Lance Armstrong's Comeback from Cancer

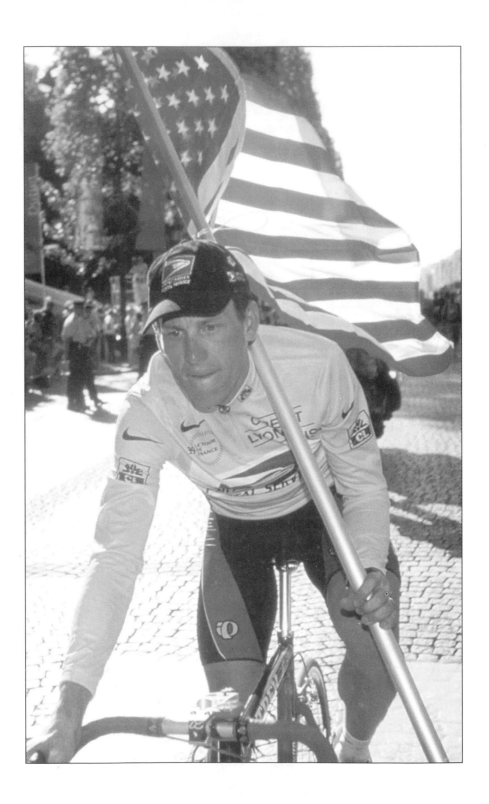

Lance Armstrong's Comeback from Cancer

A Scrapbook of the Tour de France Winner's Dramatic Career

Samuel Abt

Photographs by James Startt

Van der Plas Publications, San Francisco

Copyright © 2000 Samuel Abt
Printed in USA
First printing, 1999

Published by
Van der Plas Publications
1282 7th Avenue
San Francisco, CA 94122
U.S.A.

U.S book trade distribution
Seven Hills Book Distribution
Cincinnati, OH

Cover design
Kent Lytle, based on a photograph by James Startt
of Lance Armstrong during the second time trial
in the 1999 Tour de France.

Photography
James Startt except as marked

Publisher's Cataloging in Publication Data
Abt, Samuel
Lance Armstrong's Comeback from Cancer:
A scrapbook of the Tour de France Winner's Dramatic Career.
p. cm. Includes index.
ISBN 0-892495-25-2 (paperback original)
1. Bicycle Racing. 2. Cancer I. Authorship. II. Title.
L.C. Catalog Card Number 99-75679

This book is for Geoff Nicholson,
1929–1999,
friend, accomplice, tutor.

There are many different kinds of success,
but few of us are able to take our pick.

Ned Hanlon

There is a tide in the affairs of men,
Which, taken at the flood, leads on to fortune;
Omitted, all the voyage of their life
Is bound in shadows and in miseries.

William Shakespeare

Acknowledgments

In addition to Lance Armstrong himself, others to whom I owe thanks for their help include such riders as Frankie Andreu, George Hincapie, Tyler Hamilton, Kevin Livingston, Marty Jemison, Jonathan Vaughters, Christian Vande Velde, and Bobby Julich; such team officials as Mark Gorski, Dan Osipow, Johan Bruyneel, Johnny Weltz, Emma O'Reilly, Margot Myers, and Jim Ochowicz; such friends and traveling companions as James Startt, Becky Rast, Eric Serres, Jeremy Whittle, Stephen Ferrand, and Alasdair Fotheringham; and such colleagues as Rob van der Plas, Anne-Sophie Bolon, and my editors at the *International Herald Tribune* and *The New York Times*. As always, deepest thanks to my children, John, Phoebe, and Claire.

Introduction

This is not a biography in the usual sense, looking back at the end of a long life and its accomplishments.

At age 28, Lance Armstrong has just attained his peak as a bicycle racer; he should have many more victories to add to his record and many more rich years to spend outside the sport. Rather, this is a scrapbook of writing — brief and sometimes not so brief memories and evocations, following Armstrong from 1992, when he turned professional, to that glorious July of 1999 when he won the Tour de France. In those few years he has experienced more drama than most riders know in a lifetime, including his battle with cancer — his greatest victory.

Armstrong and I first met early in 1992 at the Tour DuPont in the United States. He was then regarded as one of the most promising American riders in years, and certainly one of the most articulate and engaging. He has remained so during his career — a considerate, accessible, and passionate spokesman for bicycle racing, and now for the conquest of cancer as well.

One of the last times we talked during the 1999 Tour de France, he proudly showed a videotape made by one of his sponsors, Nike. There on a bicycle was Armstrong, in the yellow jersey, with the words "According to cancer statistics, Lance Armstrong is not alive and riding in the Tour de France."

"Shouldn't they change 'riding' to 'winning'?" I asked. He beamed. "That's just what they're doing," he replied. Either way, his story is overwhelming, especially for those who know him as a friend. They are enormously proud of him.

Table of Contents

A Moment of Purity

What helped, of course, was that the sun came out. The same French village that can look so forlorn in the rain will glow when the sun comes out.

In any case, this was a special village, neat and tidy, picturesque even in a quiet way: the houses made of fieldstone and stucco, a town hall, school, firehouse and post office designed to be set together, and a long lawn leading to a pond with a saltbox building at the far end.

While it looked like Vermont, it was la France profonde, the heartland, on a small road in Brittany. The sign along route D81 pointed to the nearby town of Vigneux de Bretagne and the distant attractions of Nantes.

The village is called Fay de Bretagne and it is too small a place for any of the prefab shopping centers, each building a small aircraft hangar, that have been rising just outside French towns for a decade, offering parking space while underpricing the local baker and grocer.

Fay de Bretagne is too small even to have a municipal swimming pool; a notice at a bus stop gave the hours for the trip to the pool in bigger Blain up the road.

On the Rue de Solferino, named for one of Napoleon's greatest victories, a few hundred people were waiting near a banner marking the spot as a bonus sprint in the Tour de France. There were many children in the crowd, lured there by the advertising caravan that precedes the riders by an hour and flings to the spectators caps, pieces of candy, leaflets, plastic bags, little bags of sausage, giant paper hands, and supermarket flags. Adults often grapple with a child for the junk. Not in this village, though. The same decorum that marked the architecture governed the spectators.

A man at the curb explained that this was dairy country, gesturing at pastures that spread flat to the horizon. Black and white cows moved under a sky full of puffball clouds.

Where the road turns gently right, and the street name becomes the Rue de la Mairie, stands the Residence St. Joseph, an old folks' home.

About 20 residents were ranged in wheelchairs on the front lawn, facing toward the sprint banner. More than half of them were wearing either the red and yellow gas company caps or the yellow mobile phone caps that the hucksters had thrown from their cars. A few residents wore straw hats, obviously their own. Behind the line of wheelchairs, attendants in white chatted with each other.

Four old men stood on the steps leading to the residence's door.

You like the Tour de France? a visitor asked one of them. Never miss one, he said. (The bicycle race may have passed this way once before in the decade and then again may not have.) Got any favorite riders? All of them. What are you going to do after the race passes? Wait for dinner.

The noise of beeping cars and motorcycles heralded the Tour. Ten minutes later the wave of color down the road came close enough to be identified as individual riders surging toward the bonus sprint banner. The first man across the invisible line was, appropriately, the man in the yellow jersey of the overall leader. Behind him the pack formed a long unbroken line.

The riders made the soft right turn in front of the Residence St. Joseph and began heading out of the village, past St. Martin's church and homes with vegetable gardens at their sides. Already the crowd by the sprint banner had begun leaving. For them, the Tour de France had come and gone.

The four old men swiveled slowly, carefully, and watched the race pass. Like the village, the many colors of the riders' jerseys glowed in the sunlight. A mother and father came down the street, and their two small boys shrieked with joy at the disappearing riders. In that moment, it became possible to believe again in the race's purity.

Part I. Looking Back

July 25, 1999
The Man in the Yellow Jersey

Aglow in the yellow jersey of the champion, Lance Armstrong completed the final leg of his three-week journey to Paris, mounted the last of his many victory podiums, and was proclaimed the winner of the 86th Tour de France. Only the second American to win the world's greatest bicycle race, the 27-year-old leader of the U.S. Postal Service team stood solemnly with his cap off as a French military band broke into the Star-Spangled Banner just after he was given one more yellow jersey, two more bouquets, a blue vase, and a check for 2.2 million francs ($350,000).

An immense crowd watching under a blazing sun and pure sky cheered him on the avenue of the Champs-Élysées. "It's been a tough three weeks on the legs and the head," he said after he crossed the last line, well back in the pack, and just before he left the victory podium to embrace his wife, Kristin, whose face was running with tears.

Two and a half years before, the yellow jersey, vase, and flowers would have seemed to be unlikely rewards for the Texan, who was diagnosed in October 1996 with testicular cancer that had spread to his lungs, abdomen, and brain. After surgery and three months of chemotherapy, he did not return to racing until 1998 and found it impossible to convince any team except U.S. Postal Service that he was not "damaged goods," as he put it.

Since his illness, Armstrong had dedicated himself to fighting cancer, both through an educational and fund-raising foundation that he formed in his hometown of Austin, Texas, and through his inspirational victories in what he calls "the toughest sport there is."

"I relate to cancer patients," he said at the start of the 1999 Tour. "At the same time, I can relate to the families of those who didn't make it, and that's the sad thing, and probably the more emotional and motivational."

His victory was highly popular on both sides of the Atlantic. European fans who stood at the sides of the Tour's many roads universally said they knew about his comeback and were cheering for him to win both the race and his fight against cancer. In checkups every few months, he has tested clean of the disease for two years. "It is a miracle, " he said, agreeing with a description offered at a news conference. "Fifteen or 20 years ago, I wouldn't be alive, much less riding a bike or winning the Tour de France. I think it's a miracle."

Whether it was or not, his victory was certainly the result of dedication. For two years, he had said that he had something to prove: "I'm here for the cancer community," he announced when he began his comeback in 1998. "If it wasn't for them and the big question mark that was put on me and the doubt that was put in me, I wouldn't have come back. I think there's a lot to prove for a person that's been sick, that's been treated, that's recovering.

"I'm trying to prove it can be done. It's never been attempted. It's not as if there's been any standard set. It's never been attempted in an endurance-intense sport like cycling. Most people said it couldn't be done." And now he had done it.

Armstrong finished the Tour 7 minutes 37 seconds ahead of Alex Zülle, a Swiss with the Banesto team, and 10:26 ahead of Fernando Escartin, a Spaniard with Kelme, in the overall field of 141 riders remaining of the 180 who set out July 3. Of his huge deficit, Zülle lost 6:30 on the third stage when he was trapped by a crash. Armstrong, on the other hand, had good luck throughout: He had his first flat of the Tour during the mainly ceremonial final stage, when it did no harm, as it could have done during a stage in the mountains.

A talented man of strong will and focus, Armstrong dominated the 3,690-kilometer (2,290-mile) Tour from start to finish. He began wearing the race's symbol of overall leadership on July 3 when he won the short prologue. Two days later he yielded the jersey as sprinters began to monopolize the daily stages on flat territory. Then he regained it on July 11, when he crushed the field in a long time-trial, or race against the clock, and he never gave it up. After the first of two days off, he solidified his position on July 13 by triumphing with a bravado attack in the first day in the Alps. "I raced in a style that people like," Armstrong said in an interview before he won the Tour's second long time-trial on the next-to-last day of the race. "I'm aggressive. People want attacks, they want to see the boys working. I've always said that I'd rather be the guy that lights the race up and finishes second than the guy that sits back, doesn't do anything and wins."

But, he added, despite his dominance, "I don't consider myself the boss of the race. I'm just part of the event, just part of the show."

His Alpine victory over six climbs astounded rivals, observers, and fans — not only because of Armstrong's medical history but also because he was not regarded as a strong climber. He had finished only one of his four previous Tours.

Quickly the race became cloaked in an atmosphere of suspicion and rumor that originated in the 1998 Tour when the Festina team was expelled because of its systematic use of illegal performance-enhancing drugs. That scandal was followed by half a dozen others in the many countries of western Europe where bicycle racing is a sport second only to soccer.

Seeking to stem what he denounced as innuendo, Armstrong said in an interview that he "emphatically and absolutely" denied using drugs. A week later, after prominent press display of charges that a banned drug had been detected during a urinanalysis, he said that he had made a mistake in not acknowledging that he used a cortisone-based cream for a saddle sore, and that he had a medical certificate to allow its use. The UCI, the International Cycling Union, which governs the sport, ruled that his use of the salve was not doping.

The U.S. Postal Service leader had other, far more believable explanations for his success in the Tour's mountains. "I'm a strong kid," he said. "I also got my weight down."

Looking lean, he carried 158 pounds on his 5-foot-10-inch frame, some 15 pounds less than he weighed a couple of years before.

He also credited his preparation and his teammates. In May, the team and its directeur sportif, Johan Bruyneel, spent a week in the Alps and the Massif Central, riding the Tour's roads and studying their pitfalls. Armstrong then went on to ride in the Pyrenees "six or seven hours there in the rain with Johan in the car."

"It paid off," he said. "I had a lot of help from my team. When we got the jersey and said we would defend it, people thought we were crazy, they said this team isn't strong enough. They proved they're the strongest team in the race." (Traditionally, the winner of the Tour gives his big victory check to his teammates and such team workers as mechanics and masseurs.)

Of course, people said the same about Armstrong — that he was not strong enough to win the Tour. Now he had, joining only Greg LeMond, the pioneer, the first American to win the Tour, in 1986 and then again in 1989 and 1990.

Speaking of LeMond, Armstrong called him "a good friend of mine, and the greatest American cyclist ever." But his victory and LeMond's were different, he continued, because LeMond rode for French teams, while Armstrong "did it with an American sponsor and an American team, seven of the nine guys being Americans. That is, first of all, unheard of," he said. "Two years ago, people would have thought you were crazy." In its first two Tours, in 1997 and 1998, U.S. Postal Service did not win a stage. "What we did this year is a fantastic achievement for this team and for American cycling," Armstrong said. "To think about having a mostly American team — boy, that's huge."

His performance was praised by former champions. "He attacks just when you should," said Bernard Hinault, a Frenchman who won five Tours, the last in 1985. "In the Tour, we need fighters, and he's a real fighter."

Raymond Poulidor, the darling of French fans three decades ago, said, "The French admire Armstrong for the right reasons. The French always admire a man for the way he's lived his life, with courage."

Hennie Kuiper, a Dutchman who finished second in the Tour in 1977 and 1980, and later became Armstrong's directeur sportif with the former Motorola team, said, "After his illness, he's been thinking about his life and he's a lot more explosive and aggressive in his reactions. After that illness, he knows what life is. He can win everything. He will win everything. He's so strong psychologically."

Discussing his victory, Armstrong put it in a broad context: "This race and my performance here are going to affect a lot of people in a positive way, in a wonderful, fantastic way. I'm proud to be a cancer survivor and I'm proud to do this, I really am. I think I've told my story. That's what I always wanted to do. I've shared my story with the world. By winning the Tour, you stick in the hearts and minds of the cycling public. You can win every classic and the world championship, but the Tour is everything."

What does he do for an encore? Armstrong was asked. "There is nothing. If you win the Tour de France, the only thing you can do is try to win it again. That's it. Next year, I'll be here.

"I hope that next year, when I'm training and getting ready for the Tour, that I can approach it the way I did this year. That person was an outsider, who nobody expected to win the Tour. I hope I can still approach it with the same hunger."

Then it was time to celebrate, and that was some victory party for Armstrong and his U.S. Postal Service teammates. Two hundred of their closest friends and sponsors filled two rooms of the chic Musée d'Orsay a few hours after the riders took a victory lap on the Champs-Élysées as the American flag fluttered behind the man in the yellow jersey. "My baby," his mother, Linda, greeted him as he arrived at the museum.

His mother, who is what the French would call a pistol if they spoke English, was still mistaken, at age 45, for his wife. Like many others at the celebration, she had a few T-shirts she wanted him to autograph.

Everybody found a T-shirt, in fact, on the chairs at the sit-down dinner that followed the Champagne reception. It said "1999 Tour de France Champion," and had an American flag. There were also yellow caps, similarly inscribed, for each guest. "We planned to have a party for 70, but it grew," said Thom Weisel, the president of the team's management staff. The former head of Montgomery Securities, Weisel sponsored earlier in the decade the Subaru-Montgomery team that had as its goal a place in the Tour de France. When it was offered half a berth in 1993, with the other half going to the Chazal team from France, Weisel rejected the offer and vowed to be back soon with a team that would get a full share.

The rejection of an invitation was believed to be a first in the history of the Tour, which began in 1903 and has been interrupted only by world wars. "The offer is great and wonderful but disappointing," a Subaru-Montgomery official said then. "How could we share a team? How do you work with guys you don't know and have never raced with?"

Now, six years later, Weisel looked triumphant. So did Mark Gorski, the 1984 Olympic gold medalist in the bicycle sprint, who put together the present team with Dan Osipow. They hired Armstrong when there were no other takers, and now one of his new trophies — a big golden key with the names of peaks in the Alps and Pyrenees that the Tour climbed — was posed in front of a Musée d'Orsay bust of Jeanne Balzé, identified as the daughter of the painter Raymond Balzé, a student of Ingres a century and a half ago. Painted nymphs cavorted on the ceiling, and an ice sculpture of a bicycle rider slowly melted in the summer heat, dripping into a ring of pans that protected the parquet floor.

Armstrong was customarily gracious. He signed autographs, chatting with representatives of the team's two dozen secondary sponsors and posing for photographs with his wife, Kristin, who was expecting their first child. Life was very good for both of them — a few days later they would fly to the United States for a round of television and publicity appearances and a congratulatory visit to the White House.

As he said a few days before, Armstrong was puzzled to be such a celebrity. "Am I the same person?" he asked. "I think so. Anyway, I'm enjoying all this. It won't last forever, that I know. I have to know that in 10 years' time I'll be another ex-athlete. And that's fine with me. Maybe some people will remember me, but people forget. That doesn't worry me. The cause — my cancer foundation — will live on."

At the victory party he looked comfortable, surrounded by friends and well-wishers. For all his ease, however, he acknowledged that he had just spent three weeks as demanding on his mind as on his legs. "The hardest thing about being in the yellow jersey," he said during the race, "is the attention — the added attention and the commitments. You don't leave the race at the same time everybody else leaves and has a massage, a nap and an after-race meal. You're still at the protocol ceremony, medical control, press conferences. Over time, it starts to wear you out a little bit."

Additionally, Armstrong spent much of his time fending off suspicions, doubts, and innuendos about drugs.

* * *

This was the Tour of Renewal that wasn't. "We didn't quite make it," said Jean-Marie Leblanc, the Tour de France's director, shortly before the finish in Paris. "We closed a lot of back doors, but we accomplished only part of what we hoped to do." Other officials and observers agreed.

One early way to measure whether the Tour recovered luster with its millions of fans after a drug scandal the year before was to check the size of the crowds that turned out to watch the race. By that standard, the results were mixed.

Although immense numbers stood as usual at the sides of most roads, they were people through whose villages and cities the riders were passing. In other words, they merely had to step out of their homes to watch the riders glide swiftly by on the flat.

Where the crowds thinned out was where they are customarily thickest: Atop the mountain passes where diehard fans often camp for days beforehand to watch the action unfold for an hour far down from the peak. In 1999, the turnout on the fabled Galibier climb in the Alps, where fans usually pick out favorite riders' names with stones in the yearlong snowfields, was about a third that of the year before. On the ascent to Alpe d'Huez, which is usually two long lines of trailers on either side of the 21 hairpin curves, there was plenty of room. In the Pyrenees, the crowds were even sparser, with the Tourmalet climb, often before on the verge of a riot, strangely quiet. The Piau–Engaly stage was a study in bucolic calm.

So, if the spectators were there, perhaps the real fans were sitting home or at the beach, disenchanted.

They would have had much to be further disenchanted with during the 86th Tour. An atmosphere of mistrust and, as some saw it, paranoia was prevalent. "Everybody was waiting for a bomb to explode," an official of French television said, accurately.

The Tour de France was stung by the drug scandal and subsequent rider revolt against police investigatory methods the year before and, this time, it attempted to avoid trouble by having the UCI increase blood tests that hint at the use of such illegal performance-enhancing drugs as the artificial hormone EPO. The Tour also conducted its customary urinanalyses of the daily stage's winner and runner-up, the overall leader, and two riders selected at random.

To general lack of surprise, the Tour's tests caught nobody using drugs — only one rider had been detected by them in a decade. The blood tests also caught nobody even though they detected three riders, including Marco Pantani, the winner of the previous Tour, in the Giro d'Italia in May.

Did this mean the riders were clean? Not according to a segment of the press, which reckoned, probably correctly, that the riders were being more careful to beat the tests. Whatever the reason, some newspapers, especially in France, were full of daily doubts. "There are journalists in France and there are doctors on French teams who think I've been given something special by my oncologist," Armstrong said. "They think I was given drugs that boost performance.

"It's the exact opposite: I was given things that can kill you. I was given platinum. Anybody in this race wants to go have platinum, feel free. I can assure you it's not peformance-enhancing."

The use of platinum in chemotherapy was developed by one of Armstrong's two main doctors, Lawrence Einhorn, at Indiana University. His treatment is based on Cisplatin, which has been described as a novel, potent, and extremely toxic drug with severe side effects.

"That kind of talk, it makes me sick," Armstrong continued in discussing the innuendos. "But when the race is over, that stuff doesn't live. The victory and the people that I touch and the story that I can tell — that lives."

Armstrong had his own explanation for his success, and he elaborated on it: "I never focused on the Tour before, I always focused on the classics," one-day races of the spring and fall. "This event, if you want to be in the front, it has to be your focus. I always did the classics for the team, and I was a fair climber then. But at my highest level — '93, '94, '95, '96 — when was I tested in the big mountains? I wasn't. It's true. You don't get tested in the high mountains if you're a rider of the spring and fall.

"It was only last year in the Vuelta, the Tour of Spain, when that was an objective," he continued, referring to the Vuelta à España, the three-week race the previous September where his comeback began to bear results. "That was a focus, I went for it, and I was light at that point as well. It helped that I lost a lot of weight. Because of the success in the Vuelta, naturally the team, because the Tour is the biggest race for them, they wanted me to focus on the Tour. The Tour de France was never my objective before."

Somewhat bitterly, he recalled that a British journalist had questioned him that spring about his racing schedule, "needling me, 'What about Amstel? What about Liège? What about Flèche?' classics that he intended to downgrade because of his Tour training.

"I said 'I'm building up for the Tour,' and he said, sort of half-joking, 'So what are you now, a Tour rider?' With a smirk on his face.

"I didn't respond but I knew that day I was a Tour rider. I had a lot of doubts about it, but Bruyneel," who became his directeur sportif late the year before, "from day one, he was 100 percent sure of me. He sent me an e-mail last year just after the Vuelta, before the world championships. My condition was coming up and he assumed that I was going to win the world championship. He sent me a one-line e-mail that said, 'I look forward to seeing you on the podium in Paris with your rainbow jersey on.' I didn't get the rainbow jersey again," finishing fourth, "but it was a pretty good prediction. It was a strong e-mail."

Armstrong also explained his climbing skills by pointing out that he honed them almost daily when he was at his French home in Nice on the Riviera. "I climb all the time," he said. "In Nice, the only way you can get away from cars is to go uphill. On easy days, on quiet days, I climb. Because if I go down along the sea, I'd get killed by a car." (He had, in fact, been knocked off his bicycle that spring by a motorist along the shore.)

"On a hard day, when I want to do five, six, seven hours, I climb. In Nice you can do massive climbs, you can ride right into the foot-hills of the Alps. The terrain near Nice is 60 kilometers long and steep, just like anything you'll find in the Tour. It could be even harder." In sum, he said that he owed his climbing skill to "the weight loss and the fact that I simply added more climbing."

However he explained it, some suspicions refused to die. The sport had been tarnished since the previous Tour, and there were some who believed that Armstrong's victory was not credible. "I had to handle all the questions and deal with all the speculation, but it was worth it." he judged at the finish.

Laughing at the spectacle was Manolo Saiz, the directeur sportif of the ONCE team from Spain and a man whom Tour authorities tried un-successfully to ban because of what they considered his derisory atti-tude toward the race and the country. "The Tour has found a new boss to dominate the race," Saiz said midway through. "And look how he isn't allowed to enjoy his victory. The press dirties him with its sus-picions. You're dirtying not only a rider," he warned, "but also an illu-sion that nourishes millions of fans."

What Saiz did not say — or did not know — was that the illusion he referred to had nourished Armstrong himself many years before.

Part II. The First Lance

September 16, 1992
A Humble Beginning

Finishing his first bicycle race as a professional by riding so far behind that he was alone, Lance Armstrong began thinking the unthinkable. "I thought maybe I wasn't any good," he said. "I thought, 'God, these guys are that much better than me.' It was very humbling."

Armstrong was not easily humbled. On the eve of his 21st birthday, he was confident, articulate, likable, and one of the brightest prospects in the sport. But for a few weeks that summer he was simply another rider hunched over his handlebars, pumping his legs to no great, or even good, result. In a word, humbled.

As an amateur the month before, he was a favorite in the road race in the 1992 Olympic Games in Barcelona but finished out of the top 10 because, as he said, "I just didn't have the best legs. I had good legs, but other guys had better legs."

A few weeks later, after he signed as a professional with the Motorola team based in the United States, he was entered in his first pro race, the Clasica San Sebastian, a World Cup competition in Spain. The rainy weather was against him, and so was the distance — 234 kilometers (145 miles), many more than he was accustomed to as

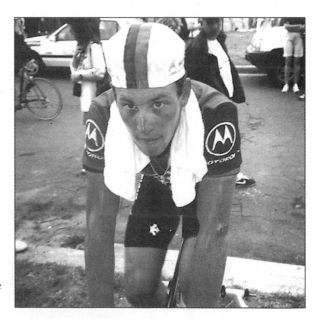

Warming up during the 1992 Tour DuPont in the U.S. as a promising amateur. He would go on to win the race twice as a professional.

an amateur. "It's tough when it's 250, 260 kilometers, but 200 I have no problem with," Armstrong said.

He finished 111th — dead last, 11 minutes behind the rider in 110th place. All alone as he plowed on, Armstrong refused to quit, as 95 of the 206 starters did. "It was my first race, my first professional race, and I didn't want to quit my first race," he explained. "I didn't want to finish, but I didn't want to quit either."

Blooded in battle, he began to do well: a stage victory in the Tour of Galicia in Spain, second place in the Championship of Zurich — another World Cup one-day race — then a victory in a small Italian race. It was an astonishingly successful start to his professional career and confirmed his promise as the heralded amateur who beat professionals to win the Settimana Bergamasca race in Italy two years before.

In mid-September 1992, Armstrong came down to earth in the Tour de l'Avenir, the Tour of the Future, a French showpiece for young and promising riders.

Although he knew that Miguel Indurain and Greg LeMond both won the Tour de l'Avenir early in their careers and thus attracted their first broad attention, Armstrong was modest beforehand about his goals in the race.

"It's sort of preparation for the rest of the season, the remaining World Cup races," he said. "I'd like to have a stage win here. Definitely. That's a goal. But the overall classification, I have to see how it goes."

By the end of the 10-day race in Brittany, Armstrong did not have a stage victory and was not so high in the standings either. Nevertheless, said his Motorola coach, Jim Ochowicz, "Lance is riding heads up, and we're very pleased. He's definitely got a winning attitude. You don't have to motivate him."

Besides attitude, Armstrong said, his form was good. "Good, but you never know, it comes and goes so quick. You get good form and there's that crest you have to hold and ride for as long as you can. It's pretty easy to go over it and start your descent."

While his form held, however, Armstrong had a full racing schedule. He was scheduled to ride next in the Tour of Ireland and then in such World Cup races as Paris–Tours, the Grand Prix of Lombardy and the Grand Prix of the Americas in Montreal. "A lot of riding," he conceded, "but I'm begging for it."

He also had an inner schedule, and it called for him to be nothing less than a great star.

Armstrong had practiced and polished the line, used it in so many interviews now that his delivery was perfect. The straight man asked the inevitable question: Are you the next Greg LeMond? "No," he answered, "I'm the first Lance," (a healthy chuckle here for punctuation) "the first Armstrong."

It reads glibber than it sounds. The adjective often attached then to Armstrong was "brash," but perhaps that was only his way of seeking self-protection. Speaking the Lance line, Armstrong could be understood to be asking for some breathing room, for respite against the LeMond comparison. Cut him some slack, as they say back home in Texas. He was still only 20 years old. "I don't think it's fair to compare me to Greg LeMond," he said earlier in the year during the Tour DuPont in America. "He's a great athlete, and I think I'm a good athlete.

"Physically, we're a lot different," continued Armstrong, who was 5 feet, 10 inches and 180 pounds to LeMond's 5-10, 152. "He's a big guy but he's not as big as me. Body type, there's no comparison. He turned pro when he was 19, but he also got married when he was 19, so I guess he started everything a little early."

Armstrong began competing on a bicycle at 12, "just to keep busy," but focused on other sports. "Being from Texas, of course I tried football, the mainstream sports thing, then tried swimming and got into triathlon from there, and then got into cycling from there."

He was honest about why he changed sports. "I wasn't any good at football. No speed, no coordination."

Swimming — 1,650 meters indoors, 1,500 meters outdoors — was no different. "Again no speed," Armstrong said.

That analysis carried over to road racing. Asked to list his weaknesses, Armstrong said, "I don't have a lot of speed in cycling either. I'm not very quick in the sprint."

For his strengths, he named climbing and time-trials. Somewhere in between his strengths and weaknesses he put bike-handling skills. "They've improved greatly," he thought. "A lot of triathletes don't have very good bike-handling skills, because they don't ride in packs."

Riding in packs offers other advantages, he continued, including the opportunity to compare yourself directly to your opponents. "The day that you're on, you're riding, and you get this feeling that's like..." The words trailed off as Armstrong searched for a way to define ecstasy.

"You're tired and you're hurting," he resumed, "but you just look around and you can tell that the guy next to you is hurting one notch more than you and you're recovering that much faster than him, and that's an incredible feeling."

Victory is another high. "When it's going good — I should say when you're winning — it's one of the most luxurious sensations. It's an incredible feeling to win major races, to come across with your hands in the air. It's like no other feeling in the world."

Victory mattered a lot to Armstrong. "I want to be a star," he said in an even voice. "I know I want to do the Tour de France, I know I want to win the Tour de France. I think I can someday get to that level, but that's a long way off, a lot of hard work. The desire is there, the ambition is there, the goal is there. It's only a matter of doing the hard work and winning the race. "Everybody wants to win the Tour de France; everybody from Category 4 up says, 'I want to win the Tour,' yet only one guy can win it each year," he continued. "LeMond has won it three times, and look at his crowds, the way he's responded to. It's amazing.

"Win the Tour de France and you're a star. I'd like to be a star. "I'm sure I'd get sick of all the pressure and all the appearances, but I'd like to try it for a while."

July 6, 1993
The Big Show

Lance Armstrong had made it to what he called "the big show, the big deal, the Super Bowl," and what everybody else calls the Tour de France.

Armstrong could be excused for his excitement because he was 21 years old and hardly anybody else in the bicycle race, including the kid who distributes soft drinks at the finish line, was even close to being that young.

"This is my style, this is what I like," Armstrong said with a beatific smile. "From what I've seen, this is my type of race." At that point, he was reminded, he had seen nothing more than the perfunctory medical examination that all riders pass through. "There you are," he replied. "Just the medical exam and all that attention, photographers, reporters, the room full of people, the electricity. It's the Super Bowl."

If Armstrong could generate that much enthusiasm for a test of his blood pressure, how would he react to the race itself? To judge from his first few days in the Tour de France, just fine.

He was one of the youngest men to start the Tour in years, along with Andrea Peron, an Italian with Gatorade, who also was 21. Because Armstrong was also a neo-pro, as first-year professionals are called, his entry caused a bit of controversy.

Miguel Indurain, then the Tour champion, was also a 21-year-old neo-pro in his debut in 1985. There was no similar controversy then because Indurain, who dropped out after four of the 21 stages, had not shown the great potential that Armstrong had. In other words, the Spaniard was regarded as cannon fodder — as Peron was — and the American was considered a star of the future if he was not misused.

The possibility of burnout troubled some observers, but not Armstrong or officials of his team.

"I'm here to learn, really," he said in an interview before the Tour started. "I don't expect anything. I don't expect to win a stage, I don't expect to take a jersey."

"But I'd like to," he added hastily. "I'd really like to win a stage. I definitely think it's possible." He acknowledged, though, that his goal was "rather lofty."

Armstrong was open about his desire to succeed. In his short career, he had won a few big races — including the U.S. professional championship the previous month and a $1 million bonus — and done well enough in others to be recognized as a major future talent.

The future was not quite now, Armstrong conceded.

For now, his plans were to race only the first two weeks of the three-week Tour. The Alps were on his calendar, but not the Pyrenees.

"We'll take it day to day," said Jim Ochowicz, the Motorola team's general manager. "We'll see how he's recuperating each day. He'll be monitored by Max Testa, the team doctor. I'd like to get Lance through the Alps, because he needs to know some of those climbs. He's never done them. You need to get through this first time to know the roads, the climbs, all the atmosphere, all the things that come with the Tour de France that you don't find at other races."

"This is a learning experience," Ochowicz said. "I definitely don't think he's too young. If I were worried about that, I wouldn't have had him here."

Armstrong was not worried either, he said as he sat in his hotel room, stripped to the waist, wearing a silver outline of the state of Texas on a chain around his neck and awaiting a rubdown. Nor, he insisted, was he intimidated. "No, no," he said quickly and predictably when asked about that.

When he was riding for the U.S. amateur team in the Tour DuPont, he admitted that his long-term goal was to win the Tour de France. Now he was putting it into broader perspective. "When you're a kid you say you want to ride the Tour, but realistically I've been thinking about it just the last couple of months," he said.

In that time he finished second in the DuPont, third in the Tour of Sweden, and first in the K-Mart Classic, the Thrift Drug Classic, and the CoreStates Championship — the so-called U.S. triple crown that earned him the $1 million bonus. (Rather than accept $50,000 a year for 20 years, the team chose a $600,000 settlement, with $210,000 taken immediately by the Internal Revenue Service. The rest was put into the team pool and Armstrong's share, still under discussion, might have amounted to no more than $30,000.)

No, Armstrong continued, he was not intimidated, but he was excited. "I feel like I'm ready," he said. "I'm not necessarily ready to make it into Paris, but that may not be in my best interest either. I'm ready to start, I'm ready to race the beginning part. I'm not even scared of the mountains. I'm looking forward to that part."

By constant practice, he had become a good climber, he felt. "When I first came into cycling, time-trialing was my forte," he said. Now the race against the clock was his weakness, one that cost him possible victory in the DuPont.

He blamed his emphasis on improving his climbing. "You work on one, you lose the other," he said. "I didn't use to be able to climb at all. If we saw a hill," and here he snapped his fingers, "I was gone. I worked so much on my climbing — always climbing, climbing, climbing — till it came around. I still have to lose some weight, though, to make it easier going up the hills." He then weighed 165 pounds. "I was a big kid when I was growing up," he said, "because I was swimming so much from a young age — 12.

"At age 13, 14, those years when your body develops and you go through so much growth, I was swimming 10,000 meters a day," he said. "That's all upper-body work, so you can imagine that when I was 14 years old I was this incredibly buffed-out little kid. Not the Hulk but definitely bulky. And I'm still trying to shed it."

A Motorola masseur was knocking on the door, and Armstrong prepared to leave for his rubdown. He had a few final words. "There's been a lot of talk: People say a 21-year-old neo-pro, putting him in the Tour..." He left the sentence unfinished.

He added: "The fact of the matter is I'm physically 100 percent right now, mentally I'm very motivated, and I want to do it. That can't be harmful. I know it's going to be tough but I'm not risking anything.

"Where guys risk burnout and the remainder of their season is in the third week, the last 10 days," he continued, "and I'm going to be gone by then. I'll get the benefits of two weeks of racing and get out before I start to kill myself."

There was absolutely, positively no chance he would continue into the grueling Pyrenees?

Armstrong thought about that. "I'd have to be in a pretty good position to stick around," he finally said. He thought about that, too. He said not another word, but the sly smile on his face said it for him.

July 12, 1993
That First Victory

Finding a perilous opening along the crowd barriers in the last 50 meters, Lance Armstrong lived out his dream by winning a daily stage in his first Tour de France. "It came down to desire," he said after he won a six-man sprint into the historic city of Verdun in northeastern France. When a narrow lane opened in the dash to the finish, he surged through, caught the leader, and crossed the line with his arms thrust high and pumping in victory.

Armstrong finished half a bicycle length ahead of Raul Alcala, a Mexican with the WordPerfect team and the only rider who finished ahead of him in the Tour DuPont in the United States in May. "An old rival," Alcala called Armstrong, sounding as if the young American had been a professional bicycle racer far longer than 10 months.

Officials hurriedly inspected the record books to see if Armstrong was the youngest to win a daily stage of the Tour. The answer was "maybe," since Henri Cornet, who won the Tour by disqualification in 1904 at age 20, either did or did not win a stage, according to different histories.

After he left the victory podium, Armstrong was as jubilant as any veteran victor in the Tour. "I'm very happy about that," he said redundantly. Then, he watched a replay of the final sprint. "There was nothing I could do," he said as he saw himself blocked while the six riders

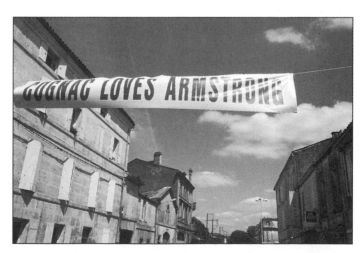

After his first victory, Armstrong became a favorite of many. This banner in Cognac on Stage 18 of the 1999 Tour is testimony to that.

dug for the line. When the leader, Ronan Pensec, a Frenchman with Novemail, swerved slightly to his left, a narrow lane along the barriers opened, and Armstrong bolted through.

He finished the 184.5-kilometer stage from Chalons-sur-Marne to Verdun in 4 hours 22 minutes 23 seconds. The main pack was 15 seconds behind the six breakaways, who got free five kilometers from the finish.

Depending on how well he did in the time-trial and then across the Alps later in the week, Armstrong would continue on a day-to-day basis, but was not expected to be allowed by his team to finish the Tour. The physical and psychological demands of the race were generally regarded as too taxing for a rider his age.

There had been no holding him back so far, though. He had contested some of the first week's sprint finishes, was a main force in Motorola's surprisingly high third-place finish in the team time-trial, and kept following breakaways toward Verdun until he found the right one. "We needed to win today," Armstrong said, citing Motorola's failure a day before, when it had three riders in a seven-man breakaway and could not place a man first.

July 17, 1993
Time to Bow Out

Lance Armstrong, who started the Tour as "a learning experience," decided before the 12th stage that school was out.

The distance, 287.5 kilometers (187.6 miles), was the longest day in this Tour. But it would have offered the boy from Plano, Texas, a few final lessons.

One was how to steal a victory. It was taught by Fabio Roscioli, an Italian with the Carrera team whose name was previously known primarily to family and friends before he won the stage by more than seven minutes. Roscioli went off alone at Kilometer 104 and built a lead of as much as 16 minutes 10 seconds as the pack refused to respond.

Perhaps it was the heat of a perfect summer's day, perhaps it was exhaustion after the Alpine ordeal the last few days, perhaps it was that Roscioli started the day in 123rd place, nearly an hour and 20 minutes behind the leader, Miguel Indurain, and was dangerous to nobody high in the standings. Or, perhaps, it was simply a collective present — a day on vacation — to Indurain on his 29th birthday.

Whatever the reason, Roscioli, who had spent his career in the shadows, fetching raincoats and water bottles for Carrera leaders, held on to win by 7 minutes 14 seconds and moved up to 70th place overall. It was the first known victory for the Italian, who would turn 28 a few days later, since he became a professional in 1987.

Roscioli had no plans for the long breakaway, he explained later. "I just saw the chance and went."

The stage began with Jim Ochowicz of Motorola announcing that "Lance is not here for the start today. Lance is done, he's finished today. He's going by car to his home in Italy.

"It was time. This morning, when he woke up, his blood pressure was a little bit off, his pulse was up, and it was time to say, 'Hey, Sayonara,' to this.

"He reached his goals," Ochowicz said. "He got a lot of experience out of his 12 days in the Tour de France, so he's leaving in a very positive mood."

Armstrong said the same before the start of the second of two demanding stages in the Alps.

Referring to his victory in a stirring sprint finish in Verdun, he said, "I'm still learning, but I've already accomplished everything I want to do. I'm not going to push myself too much today," he went on. "If I feel like I'm digging a hole, then I'm going to retire myself from the race."

He struggled through the Alps, describing the first stage, 204 kilometers, as "too long and too cold," after he finished 86th, nearly 22 minutes behind the winner. The second day he was 97th, nearly 29 minutes behind, after 180 kilometers more. That dropped him to 62nd place overall from a high of 12th after his stage victory.

He also experienced the frustration that marks struggling riders: He was so far behind at the end of the second day in the Alps that his team car was no longer waiting for him at the finish line in the mountaintop resort of Isola 2000 and he had to ride his bicycle yet a few more miles up a dusty gravel trail to his hotel. "As if the stage wasn't enough, we have to climb this thing," he grumbled, expletive deleted, in what amounted to his farewell address to the 80th Tour de France.

So he missed out on one of the loveliest stages in the last few Tours, traversing the bottom of the Alps and their barren canyons before turning right above Nice and passing through the fertile backlands of the Provence.

In its indolent way, the pack might have been sightseeing all the way from the start in the Italianate village of Isola, with its umber and pale green walls glowing in the sun, and then through Vence and Grasse, past the Chagall chapel, past palm, cypress, and olive trees, past laurel bushes ablaze with pink, white, and red flowers. What a change this was from the fields of weathered boulders and patches of dirty snow in the Alps.

Then came long, long kilometers of fields planted in wine grapes for Côtes de Provence, an inexpensive and genial rosé, and Côteaux Varois, ditto but red. Even the finish into the Mediterranean port of Marseille offered some uplifting views of the sea.

Armstrong will get many more chances to enjoy the Tour's vistas. "He's definitely got the fight to be a top rider," Ochowicz said. "He left here knowing he's got to work a little bit on his time-trialing and his climbing. In the other stages, he can handle that. He's already well ahead of the game there."

Aug. 29, 1993
World Champion

Battling back after two crashes in the rain, Lance Armstrong surged ahead about halfway into the final lap and held on to win the men's professional road race in the World Cycling Championships in Oslo.

He covered the 257.6 kilometers (159 miles), in rainy and cold conditions that made the road slippery, in 6 hours 17 minutes 10 seconds, for an average speed of 40.9 kilometers an hour. Miguel Indurain of Spain edged Olaf Ludwig of Germany in a sprint for second place. Both riders finished 19 seconds behind Armstrong.

Armstrong said he tried to be patient and control himself "because I knew it would happen on that last lap."

"The wet road was difficult," he said. "I crashed twice during the race. There were guys crashing all around me. Of course, I didn't want to get a gap and crash on the last lap. But it seemed that every time you were careful you fell over."

Armstrong was in fourth place when the last lap started and made his winning move on the last big climb, quickly building an 18-second lead. "When I got with the leaders, they were not organized," he said. "No one was working and the situation was totally

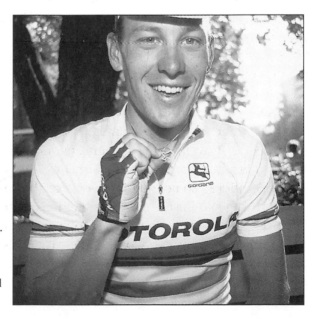

If Armstrong is superstitious, it's about his Texas State necklace. Since his early days as a professional, this prize jewel has always danged from his neck.

negative. I did not want to go too fast, but once I opened a gap that was it.

"I just went all out on the climb," he added. "I realized I had it won with about three kilometers to go. I looked back and I didn't see anybody.

"At that point I didn't believe it. To be honest, I still don't believe it."

Indurain, who led briefly with about 25 kilometers left, said he almost had to withdraw at the midway point of the race. "I wasn't feeling very well," Indurain said. "I was about to get off the bike. It was very tough in lap 7 and 8. I started to feel better toward the end. I kept riding, and I had enough power for the sprint."

The severity of more than six hours' riding in bitter conditions was illustrated by the fact that only 66 finished out of 167 starters.

Indurain described the course as "very dangerous."

"I began the race carefully because of that, but it was hard, and so cold," he said. "I was feeling strong toward the end, and I knew that I would be good for the sprint. To win the title is another thing. It always will be difficult to break away, because someone is always watching me."

Armstrong became only the second American to win the pro road race, and one of the youngest winners ever. Greg LeMond was 22 years, 2 months when he won the first of his two titles in 1983. Armstrong would turn 22 in three weeks.

March 14, 1994
Team Leader

One photographer was up a ladder with a camera and another was walking around with a light meter, calling out numbers as he scanned members of the Motorola bicycle team. They were posed in front of a disused roadside chapel in Tuscany. In 1993, the team photograph had been taken in a warehouse for a high-tech look, and so — yin and yang — the next year the goal was something picturesque, even touristic. "But elegant," one of the photographers explained.

Center front among the 18 riders, the four team officials, four or five bicycles, and a team car stood Lance Armstrong.

He deserved the position of honor: Armstrong was the team leader and he wore the rainbow-striped jersey of the world's professional road-race champion. In his first full season as a professional the year before, he won the world championship, a stage of the Tour de France, the U.S. professional championship, and a $1 million prize by finishing first in a series of American races.

Winners stand center front.

Then why, in the warehouse photograph taken early the year before, when Armstrong had appeared as a professional in just half a dozen races, was he also center front? "I was the team leader a little bit last year," the Texan said in the Italian village of Castagneto Carducci, where his team was holding a training camp. "I was certainly the team leader at the Tour DuPont and throughout the million-dollar saga. In the Tour de France I had days where I was considered the man."

That didn't wash. All those races took place months after the photograph. Who knew so early that Armstrong had such star quality? He smiled broadly and ducked his head in mock humility. If anybody knew, Armstrong knew. "I was always worried about not failing," he said. "I wanted to win, but more than that, I didn't want to fail. And," he spoke slowly now, "I don't think I have."

He was determined, he continued, not to fail while he was world champion. "Over the last few years, people seem to think the rainbow jersey has had a curse upon it," he noted. The 1990 world champion, Rudy Dhaenens of Belgium, never won another race and had retired from the sport. The 1991 and 1992 champion, Gianni Bugno of Italy, had failed to win a major race the previous two years.

Armstrong hoped to end that spell soon — as early as the first classic of the spring, the long race from Milan to San Remo in Italy. "It's a big goal for me, because it's the first big race that anybody's paying attention to, and I've heard so much talk about world champions wearing the rainbow jersey and not being able to perform in the jersey. This is going to be an event where I can showcase not only my talent but the possibilities of the rainbow jersey winning a big one. "As a champion, you have to represent yourself and your team and your sponsor well, but with the rainbow jersey, you're also representing the sport and the jersey itself. With that comes added pressure tenfold."

How much of that added pressure tenfold was he feeling? "None," he said flatly.

When he first began making a name for himself as a member of the U.S. national amateur team four years before, Armstrong was sometimes regarded as arrogant. Then he started fulfilling his promise by winning races and what seemed arrogant became brash. As a professional, what seemed brash became confident, ebullient, even charming and honest. "There's no pressure, because I'm prepared," he explained. "I'm ready. I've said that all along in my career — I've always said I'm ready, I'm ready, I can do this, and I'm confident. "Now I truly feel I'm secure with myself and my career. I realize I can have success. I know it's right there. It's not anything I'm worried about. It's just a matter of going out and doing it. I still have the desire to do it, like I've always had, but now I know in my heart and my mind that I can conquer this sport and that I can conquer the races."

He had felt pressure, though. "Not from the team and not from the sport, not from my friends and not from my family. But I felt a little pressure from myself because it seems I demand a little more from myself than others do."

At 22 the second youngest man to be world champion, Armstrong also appeared to be a little more worried about his reception in the rainbow jersey than he should have been. He confessed that he sensed a certain resentment among riders on other teams. "Maybe 'resentment' is too strong; maybe I'm looking at it in a pessimistic way and I shouldn't," he said. "I'm sure there are people who are jealous."

Yet, with the season just opening, he had not been in contact with many other riders. That did not dissuade him as he hinted at an unexpected insecurity. "Surely, they're a little bit jealous," he said again of other riders. "I think most of them are thinking maybe it was a fluke, thinking it was a little bit lucky."

He did not agree. "I don't think it was lucky. I rode a great race."

Armstrong was reminded that no less a racer than Miguel Indurain, the winner of the previous three Tours de France and the second-place rider in the world championship, said afterward that Armstrong deserved the victory because he was obviously the strongest man that day. "Not everybody has the class of Indurain," he replied.

He remembered when he knew he had won: "When I turned around, four or five kilometers to go, and just saw nobody. I turned around and didn't see anybody and the last split I heard was about 20 seconds. I couldn't believe it. I thought, 'Oh my God, I'm going to win the world championship.' Then I thought, 'Oh no, I've got another lap, because this is too good to be true.' I said to myself, 'How am I going to know? I don't want to cross the line and keep going.'

"It was all starting to happen so fast. From that point on, it just all happened so quick. I said, 'I'll check the computer,' and I did and it said 250 and I said, 'Oh my God, this is it.' And I thought, 'Hopefully, the computer isn't wrong.'"

It wasn't. He won the 257 kilometer race in Oslo by 19 seconds, a big lead, and ended up by blowing kisses to the crowd. "To everybody, everybody there, the fans, the spectators. And they liked it. Before I was blowing kisses, they were sitting down and afterward they were standing up. You have to please the fans. That's part of my idea about cycling: It's a sport, it's entertainment, sports are entertainment. You can win and not be entertaining, but I think people leave a race with a better image of the sport if it's entertaining. I'm here not just to do things for myself and Motorola but to promote the sport. I want people to leave and say, 'Hey, I can't wait to go to another bike race.'"

After the race, officials tried to take the new champion to meet the king of Norway, but Armstrong refused to go along unless his mother, who often watched him race in Europe, could come too. "She was thrilled, she was thrilled for me."

At each of many checkpoints, he had to argue security men into allowing his mother to pass through. "They kept saying only the winner can come, but I told them, 'If she's not coming, I'm not coming.'"

Finally they were in a room where she watched her son shake hands with a king.

That was a long way from Texas, where Armstrong grew up as the fatherless child of a 17-year-old girl whose husband left when the boy was three. "Were we poor?" he asked, repeating a question. "No, but I certainly didn't have a silver spoon."

Had it been a long time since he had contact with his father? "Forever," he answered. "She's been remarried not that long ago, but she's been with her husband quite a long time and she loves him and I know he loves her and I care a lot for him and that's all that matters. She's happy and I'm happy. As far as I'm concerned, biology doesn't matter."

Usually a man of many words, Armstrong used just one when asked if his mother had been supportive. "Very," he said.

"It means more to me than just having her at a race," he continued. "It gives me the opportunity to spend time with her before the race or after the race, allowing her the opportunity to spectate the race. It's not a normal relationship anyway, being that she's young and she had me very young and she grew up at the same time I was growing up and we sort of grew up as friends and not as mother and son. So I grew up as one of her friends and when I'm not there all the time she really feels…" He thought about it. "Lonely " he decided.

Loneliness, any sort of unhappiness, troubled Armstrong. "I'm looking for cycling to make my life, I'm not looking for cycling to ruin my life. For some people it's certainly ruined their life or made it miserable. I've seen some cyclists that just don't appear very happy. That's the last thing I want.

"I want to be happy, I want cycling to make me happy, I want it to make my family happy and right now it's doing that. The day it doesn't is the day I'm going to stop."

A contributing factor to his happiness was the big money he began earning once he won the world championship; one report said his salary had risen tenfold to $750,000 a year.

"Everybody likes money," he said strongly. "There's nothing wrong with money. There's nothing wrong with using money as a motivation. It should be a motivation not only for athletes but for everyday people. In America, people look badly on money and don't consider it an incentive, which it is. I'm supermotivated by money. I'm not going to sit here and say money doesn't mean anything to me, because it means a lot. And I enjoy giving it back. As much as I enjoy getting money, I love to give money. Christmastime, obviously a time you give and get, I don't really care to get anything, I've got everything I ever wanted, but I like to give away stuff."

That was consistent with what he described once as his religious beliefs: "I believe in my responsibility to be a good person. I think at the end of the day, we're judged upon that. I think we're all obligated as people to be true and honest and correct."

Discussing his prospects, he was optimistic about his form and opportunities in the coming season. "I'm learning more and gaining more as far as tactics are concerned," he judged. "In the past I've been very aggressive and sometimes overly aggressive and I regret it. Certainly. But sometimes you make some mistakes when you're aggressive. I recognize those mistakes and won't make them again. So my style may appear to change but it will have the same aggression with a little more intelligence."

After more than a month of tune-up races, mainly in Italy, he would get his chance to convince doubters — real or imagined — in the first World Cup classic, Milan–San Remo. It was a special race to him because its distance, 297 kilometers (184 miles), suits a rider with his strength, aggression and stamina and because he was near the front the previous year until the final climb up the Poggio Hill, where he faded.

Armstrong explained that he had not ridden his own race then but had been working for a teammate, Max Sciandri, who had since moved from Motorola. "I was left a chance to take any opportunity, if something happened to him or he was having a bad day. At the finish, I was definitely working for him because he was there and he was feeling good and he wanted help." Sciandri finished third, Armstrong 22nd.

In 1994, the team would work for Armstrong. "I have a great relationship with this team," he said. "I count them as my friends, my best friends. And they look at me the same way. The neat thing is that the way they act toward me and the way I act toward them hasn't changed a bit. I'm still the same person with a different jersey."

As a leader, he continued, his big job was to motivate. "Head up troops," he said. "I like to think I'm a motivator. I get supermotivated myself and I feel that I can motivate. We're all on the same level here, so it's very easy for them to relate to me, to see when I'm hurting. They see when I want something, when I want to win it even if I don't tell them.

"Sometimes I tell them, sometimes I say some things in the races and I think it gets them psyched up — how great I'm feeling or how I'm going to win. Within a race I can boldly predict to my teammates, 'Hey, I'm going to win today, guys.' Before a stage or during. I think they like that. Certainly, that's a little bit confident but I think if you're saying it within the team, it's a little different than if you're blurting it in headlines. But it motivates the guys.

"Another thing that motivates them is that when they have worked for me, have sacrificed for me, the majority of the time I've come through. So when it comes around the next time and I say, 'Come on guys, we've got to chase, do some work here, I need some help,' these guys are 100 percent willing to do it because they know if anybody is going to come through for them, it's going to be me.

"And the day I can't do that is the day I need to stop racing. I don't want to let anybody down. And that's part of my motivation, that when I say, 'OK guys, let's work,' they get up there and they're on the front hammering, chasing down somebody, leading me out.

"I see these guys hurting, I see the salt forming on their shorts, I see them sweating, I hear them breathing and that motivates me.

"I'm willing to sacrifice for them. I've shown in the past that I'm willing to work for somebody else if I'm not riding well. That's not a problem. I've displayed that and I'll continue to do that. Nobody thinks that a rainbow jersey can ride on the front for his teammates, but I don't have a problem with that. If I was in a position where I had to work for somebody else, sure."

April 27, 1994
Report Card

Surrounded by team officials and teammates happy to give him guidance, Lance Armstrong appeared not to have been listening, so great was his zeal to do well in Milan–San Remo. Or did nobody point out that he was overdoing his training? All through March, in minor races in Spain and Italy, he worked hard at overdoing it: He would finish that day's long race and then go off on his own for 60 or 80 kilometers more.

Anybody who remembered him in training camp in Tuscany — moving out of his seat and nearer the television set whenever a videotape of the previous year's Milan–San Remo was playing — would understand. The rest of the team lounged in the back of the dining hall, maybe looking at the videotape, maybe not, because they had seen it so many times already. Armstrong never had enough of it: He would stand silent as the images of the race flickered by.

To no effect. "Milan–San Remo, that was a failure," he admitted later in the spring. "I give myself an 'F' there." Had he been over-

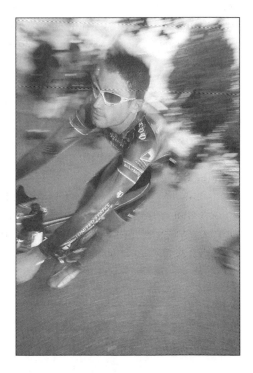

Long-time teammate George Hincapie. He played an important role in some of Armstrong's victories.

trained? "Yes," he replied flatly. "I was tired, rundown, overtrained to a point. Anyway, that was no good," he continued, brushing the race aside and rushing ahead in his review of his performances in the spring classics. The world champion had not gotten off to the impressive start he sought.

"Then Flanders, another failure, the same problem, the same feeling, the same rundown, tired feeling. Then I went to Pays Basque and that's when I started to think it couldn't get any worse. I was feeling so bad. We had a climb and I couldn't elevate my heart rate and I went straight to the back.

"After three or four days, I stopped and went home to my Italian base in Como and said to myself, 'This is the bottom. It can't get any worse than this. I have to start turning this around.' So I rested, just rested and rested. I rested a lot. I had rested before Flanders also, but it wasn't enough. After I quit Pays Basque, I rested for at least a wee." The long rest began to help him recover.

"I rode, but very minimal, saw the doctor a lot, and was feeling better, and things started to come around. I had some personal problems too that I straightened out," a reference to a former girlfriend who could not adapt to the move from Texas to Italy. For all his worldliness and suavity — a word not often applied then to Armstrong, but accurate — he was still just 22 and not that long removed from the turmoil and torments of a teenager.

"Another thing is I changed my position on my bike," he went on. "Last year I rode one position and then I went to a steeper position and then, just before Liège–Bastogne–Liège, I went back to the old position and the same bike I rode at the world championships. So I straightened out the personal problems, straightened out the position problem and things started to come around. Got my mom over, so three things at once."

Results started to come in the classics: second place in Liège, 13th in the Amstel Gold Race. "Liège was a success, that was a nice one — 'A minus.' Amstel I felt good. I would grade it on how I felt so I would give it an 'A.' Overall, it was an average spring."

Now that his results were better, Armstrong realized he had a lot to be pleased about. One was how much easier he found living in Europe in his second year there. In addition to working out the traditional problem of being an American racer in Europe, far from home and a familiar culture, he was learning more about who he was and who he hoped to become.

After he dropped out of the 1993 Tour, he returned home to Italy to recover while the race headed toward Paris. On the next-to-last day, he rejoined the race as a spectator at the final time-trial.

The real reason, he confided, was that he did not want to miss the Motorola team's traditional celebration party at a Tex-Mex restaurant in Paris. "A Texas boy like me wouldn't miss a time like that," he said.

Looking fit and relaxed at the time-trial's start south of Paris, Armstrong summed up that year's Tour with a tribute to the winner, Miguel Indurain: "He dominates. He's definitely the best bike racer around. I look at him as the ultimate."

Then he paid a meaningful personal tribute to the Spaniard. "If I came close to idolizing anybody, it would be Indurain. I'd love to ride with a guy like that. He's got a super attitude. He's not obnoxious, he's quiet, he respects the other riders, he never fusses. He's so mild-mannered. I really like him." So much so that Indurain seemed to have become a role model for Armstrong, who confessed, "I still have a temper and an attitude, sometimes.

"I wouldn't mind molding myself into his sort of character," he concluded. "Really quiet, just goes about his business."

May 8, 1994
A Change of Heart

Somewhere on the Tour DuPont's long road from Wilmington, Delaware, to Winston-Salem, North Carolina, the public changed sides, crossing over from Greg LeMond to Lance Armstrong.

The next era in American bicycle racing edged closer. It may have been a few months too early for anybody to cry, "The king is dead, long live the king" — the Tour de France should help determine how true that was — but for now the 22-year-old Armstrong ranked no lower than prince regent. That's the fellow who rules during the absence or infirmity of the nominal sovereign.

How infirm LeMond, 32, was remained a question.

"I'm feeling good, I think I'm getting it back," he insisted in an interview early in the Tour DuPont, which ended in the hush-puppy belt of North Carolina. His allergies were under control, LeMond added, and his chronic fatigue was lessened.

But there was no question about his absence. The three-time winner of the Tour de France was never a player during the DuPont: 22nd place overall, laggard finishes in both time-trials, and struggles in the mountains. At the end, he was 10 minutes 39 seconds behind the winner, Slava Ekimov of the WordPerfect team.

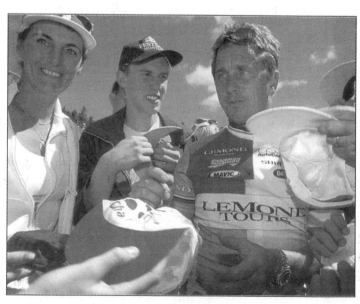

Years later, Greg LeMond would lead cycle tours and stop by the Tour de France with his guests, as in this photo taken during the 1998 Tour.

LeMond's only consolation, he said, was that "maybe this is a good sign because I've always done well in the Tour de France when I've done badly in the DuPont." And vice versa. He had not done well in the Tour de France, or any other race, since 1992, when he won the DuPont.

People were beginning to notice, even in the United States, where professional bicycle racing attracts scant attention.

When the 12-day DuPont began in Wilmington early in May, LeMond monopolized fan interest. At the short prologue to the race, Armstrong went barely noticed in his rainbow-striped jersey of the world road race champion as he pedaled to the start, passing the team car in which LeMond awaited his turn.

The car was surrounded by spectators, many of them carrying cameras and some of them carrying children. Everybody wanted a memory of LeMond. As he moved to the start line, the streets of Wilmington rang with cheers, which were renewed when LeMond finished fifth in the prologue.

Armstrong, meanwhile, was 25th on a cold and rainy evening.

"I rode like a grandma," he admitted ruefully, meaning he had been far too cautious about crashing on a stretch of wet cobblestones. A few days later Armstrong rode better, finishing third in a demanding time-trial over two big climbs. "It was tough," he said, "but I was able to push myself and it felt good to push myself."

LeMond lost more than 4 minutes on that stage and said he had been shocked at its difficulty. He slid far down the standings and remained there.

They love a winner in the United States, or at least a contender. The public turned out in gratifying numbers at the sides of the DuPont's roads through Virginia and North Carolina and at its daily small-town starts and finishes. What these fans read about in their newspapers and saw on their television was no longer LeMond but Armstrong, and their allegiance shifted from one American to the other.

The script was perfect for people who turned out to cheer "USA, USA" as the pack went by: Armstrong, a Texan, working to overtake Ekimov, a Russian. This typecasting became even more pointed as Ekimov stayed on Armstrong's rear wheel and rode defensively, refusing to attack but following each attack by his rival.

The public didn't know it, but that is the way races are won.

"To say it doesn't bother me, I'd be lying," Armstrong said. "But that's just the way the sport is."

Tell that to newspapers and television more accustomed to reporting on stock car racing: The daily theme became Ekimov as a somehow unfair shadow of Armstrong's.

"The guy in second place," said Armstrong, referring to himself, "looks like the champion now, he looks like the fighter, he looks like the guy who deserves to win. And the guy in the leadership role, he looks like he's just sucking wheel."

If the first part of the DuPont had belonged to LeMond, the second part, when the real racing began, belonged to Armstrong. After all, he was the contender.

In the mornings, when fans are allowed to wander the staging area and ask the riders for autographs, it was Armstrong's team car that was surrounded. Although LeMond continued to attract the public, too, it was obvious who won the loudest cheers at the daily sign-in and introduction.

Armstrong ended his race by holding on to second place, 1:24 behind Ekimov, with a good performance in the time-trial into Winston-Salem.

"I'm disappointed, I'm not overly happy," he said, to finish second two successive years. Armstrong promised to be back to try for victory in the DuPont the next year.

"I'm still young and inconsistent," he admitted. "I'm moving up in the ranks. I can get better."

July 2, 1994
Back at the Show

Just finished with the Tour de France's perfunctory medical examination, Lance Armstrong was sitting at a table, reading a magazine, and in a sour mood.

What had the doctors said? "They said I could start," he responded with an empty laugh. Had they said he could finish? "I'll say that. It depends on my legs and my body. It may not be in my best interest. Last year it was the first 10 days, and then it was day to day. Maybe it'll be longer than that this year. I don't want to jeopardize the second half of my season just to finish the Tour de France."

Something was bothering him. Perhaps it was the hurry-up-and-wait atmosphere in the huge convention hall in Lille where the 81st Tour de France was going through its paperwork. A year before he had been thrilled by everything about the race, including the medical examination. This time he appeared to be blasé. Perhaps he was trying not to show that he felt any pressure about being the world champion in a race that he was certainly not going to win and probably not even going to finish. Considering his age and the fact that he would defend his world championship a month after the Tour, a withdrawal before the last, grueling week in the Alps seemed sound. And yet, the man with the rainbow jersey might have been expected to ride as long as he could and as hard as he could.

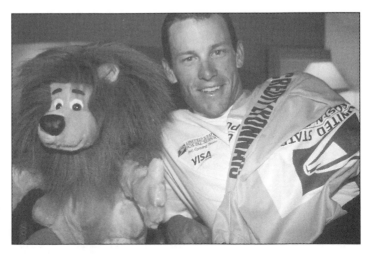

Happy to be in the Tour in 1994, who would guess some day he'd be wearing the Yellow Jersey, as he is here in 1999.

"It's not my first race as the world champion," Armstrong pointed out somewhat testily. "I had the first part of the season to get used to that responsibility.

"It seems to be much more difficult this year for some reason," he continued. "There's a lot of guys that go much faster this year. I'm just as fit and feel as good as I did last year, but my strength within the peloton has sort of gone down. A lot of riders are stronger." He did not know it then, but 1994 is now generally regarded as the beginning of the era of EPO, the illegal artificial hormone that enhances performance by multiplying the red blood corpuscles that carry oxygen to exhausted muscles. Italian teams especially are now believed to have started to use the drug that year. Although he knew none of this specifically, Armstrong suspected something.

"It's harder to race this year, cycling is harder now," he said. "In a year, I tell you, man. I hate to point fingers, and I'm not going to do that, but there are a lot of guys who are a lot better and a lot faster than last year.

"I think I can do better in the Tour," he decided. "If I can show some improvement in the time-trials and the climbs and we can do well in the team time-trial, that's successful for me. Those big climbs in the long, high mountains, I can't compete yet." But he was hopeful of becoming a better climber. "A few years ago, if we rode a 2 percent grade, I was off the back. When I was an amateur, I was a terrible climber. But I improved in that and lost weight and now I can climb fairly well. So I may be continuing to rise. It's coming naturally."

July 11, 1994
Everybody's Watching

The Curse of the Rainbow Jersey sounded like the title of a novel Lance Armstrong might read during a bicycle race, but it wasn't. He insisted that it was autobiography.

Since he won the rainbow-striped jersey in Oslo the August before, Armstrong had problems winning again in Europe. Everybody knew who he was now, he said accurately, and nobody would let him make an unaccompanied attack in a race.

"This's always going to attract attention," he said, referring to his jersey. It travels in a crowd, and so Armstrong did again in the Tour de France's eighth of 21 stages, a 218.5-kilometer (135.7-mile) slog from Poitiers to Trelissac in the Perigord region of southwestern France.

He finished 53rd among the 176 riders in the 81st Tour. Armstrong had been racing strongly enough to rank in eighth place overall, 42 seconds behind the leader, but had not been able to come close to a stage victory.

"It's so much harder to race with this," Armstrong said earlier, plucking at the jersey. "Even if you're bad in that jersey, they're going to follow your every move. Because of that jersey.

"It just sticks out, it sticks out to the eye. People assume it's dangerous."

In fact, Armstrong was dangerous and had been since he turned professional right after the 1992 Olympic Games in Barcelona.

But few opponents realized at first how strong a rider the Texan was. When he won a clutch of races in the United States, it was far, far from European notice. In his debut in the Tour de France, he slipped away in a small attack and finished first, confirming his talent. Then, on a rainy day in Norway, he broke away from the pack toward the end of the world championship road race and cruised across the line, blowing kisses to the vast crowd. King Harald presented him the jersey — and the curse that often accompanies it.

Armstrong knew that he would not win this Tour and probably would not finish it, avoiding the Alps to save his strength for the world championships on Sicily late the next month.

His goals, he said, were to win a stage and "show some improvement in the time-trials and the climbs."

The climbs would have to be in the Pyrenees, which came before the Alps. "The last week, in the Alps," Armstrong said, "I'm pretty sure I'm not going to do it."

As for time-trials, he would see soon whether he was improving. The 64-kilometer race against the clock was, Armstrong said, "a little bit long for me. I've never done a time-trial that long. I feel I have good form, so I'm interested to see where it puts me compared to last year," he continued.

He finished 27th then, 6:04 behind the winner, Miguel Indurain.

"I'm starting two minutes ahead of Indurain this time," Armstrong noted, "so I'd better go fast. I've got to go really fast" or risk being overtaken, passed, and embarrassed in the rainbow jersey. (Which was just what happened).

October 3, 1994
The Old Jersey

Lance Armstrong was back in his team jersey, a blue and red one, and only the discreet multicolored stripes at the neck and sleeves indicated that he ever wore the broad bands of the rainbow jersey.

"My new old jersey, yeah," he said of the blue and red one. Armstrong, who at the age of 21 became the second-youngest man ever to win the professional road championship, finished seventh the next August in the same race.

"I was pleased with my race," he said. "I was outnumbered a bit: When it came down to 20-odd guys, there were seven Frenchmen and seven Italians."

He was the only American left among the leaders in the race, which is the only one all season contested by national, instead of commercial, teams.

"There's not a whole lot you can do in that scenario," he added.

So, when Luc Leblanc, a Frenchman, pulled on the rainbow jersey in Sicily, Armstrong returned to the standard uniform of his Motorola team.

His feelings were decidedly mixed. All season he noted that he was closely shadowed by his rivals and never allowed to attack without drawing a crowd. Now that he was simply another rider in the pack, he felt the loss.

"I miss it," he said before the start of the Paris–Tours race, speaking of the rainbow jersey. "I realize now what I had. But I'm also realistic and I realize that nobody can wear that jersey every year. If I have one year without it, I have to do my best to regain it.

"When I won the jersey it was a surprise," he added, "and I took it and wore it for a year and you don't realize at a young age, at an early point in your career, what you have. Then when you lose the jersey, you see another person wearing it, you realize exactly what it was that you achieved. And what an honor it was.

"This whole year I knew that I was the world champion and that it was a big deal to wear the rainbow jersey," Armstrong said. "It means more now. I'm looking forward to going for it again."

Implicit in his remarks was his confidence that there would be a next time and that he would master the pressures of being world champion. He rarely complained about the responsibilities of doing well in the rainbow jersey, but it was obvious that he felt them.

"You put it down on paper and '93 was a much better year," he admitted. "Looking at it on paper. Because I had a stage victory in the Tour de France and the world championship, and those are two big accomplishments. And I didn't do that this year."

His best results in 1994 were second places in the Liège–Bastogne–Liège and the San Sebastian classics, second place in the Tour DuPont, and the strong seventh place in the world championship.

"I'm happy with my results," he continued, "but some of the results just don't stick out. Not as much as last year. I feel I performed well in the jersey, fairly consistent. My goal was to be successful in the World Cup and I'm in a good position there now."

He ranked fifth overall in the season-long series of World Cup one-day races, before Paris–Tours, in which he finished behind the leaders. Armstrong trained hard for the 250-kilometer (155-mile) race from the town of St. Arnoult en Yvelines, deep in the boondocks outside Paris, to Tours in the Loire Valley. Long, flat and windy, the race often ends in a mass sprint, as this one did, and that was not his specialty.

"I did good training for this race, and I'm extremely focused," he said beforehand. As for his form, "I think it's good."

He had one more major race on his European schedule, the Tour of Lombardy, before returning home to Texas and a busy off-season.

"I'll be busier this winter than last year," he said. "Off-the-bike stuff." Among other projects, he was helping the U.S. Cycling Federation start a program to develop younger riders and he expected to work as a spokesman for organizations fighting multiple sclerosis.

Also he had an appointment at a concert with the Rolling Stones, some of whom are bicycle racing fans. "That's exactly right, Nov. 5 in San Antonio," Armstrong said. "I'll get up on stage and jam with the boys a little bit. Then the 6th, 7th and 8th I have to be in San Francisco for a multiple sclerosis convention."

He said that nobody close to him had the neurological disorder but that he hoped to raise funds for research as a good citizen. "I've always been one," he said. "It's serious stuff that I do out of my own time and for absolutely nothing."

He would continue to train, of course, looking forward to the next season, especially the next world championship, which would be held in Colombia.

"I've got to be realistic and not expect to win that race every year," he repeated. "It's OK, I'm happy. But I tell you now, I'll be much hungrier before Colombia than I was before Sicily."

July 4, 1995
Stirrings of Ambition

At the start of a new Tour de France, Lance Armstrong was ready, willing and, he hoped, able. About able, he would know in a few weeks. About ready and willing, he had no doubts.

"I'm definitely fit, much more fit than I've ever been in my life, ever," he said. "I feel better, I feel stronger, my tests are better, and my head is great.

"I'm extremely motivated, certainly more motivated for this Tour than I've ever been," he continued before the start of the 82nd Tour de France. This was the third Tour for the 23-year-old leader of the Motorola team and the first he expected to finish.

"I think I have a better understanding of the Tour de France now and how grand it is and what it truly means to the sport and to the sponsors and the people," he said. "I've never been as excited about the Tour de France."

Experience was the difference in his attitude, rarely before considered blasé.

"The first year, OK, I may have been excited," he admitted. "But I had no clue, no idea what I was coming into. Last year," when he wore the rainbow jersey and was a marked man, unable to come close to his stage victory in his Tour debut, "I may have been a bit disillusioned.

"Now I realize what the Tour de France is about: the biggest spectacle in the sport. Cycling in July is the biggest sport in Europe. It's the ultimate in July and a great place to shine."

Armstrong intended to shine. Yes indeed.

"This year I have some goals in mind and I'm going to be fighting," he announced. "First and foremost, I have to finish the race. I want to win a stage — the team has to win a stage."

Motorola, which was based in the United States but had a multinational roster, had not won a stage in the Tour since Armstrong triumphed at Verdun not quite midway in the 1993 Tour. But the Texan thought his team had an excellent chance in the time-trial between Mayenne and Alençon. Third in the team time-trial two years before and second the previous year, Motorola, he promised, would go all out.

But back to personal goals: "I want to ride strongly in the time-trials and the mountains. And if that all adds up to — I don't know what that adds up to in the end."

Of course he did. Less freewheeling than he was a few years ago, just as likable, Armstrong finally came out with it.

"If I'm super, super, super, I can maybe hope to finish in the top 10. I don't know what 10th place is, normally about 20 minutes behind. If you're riding strongly in the time-trials and don't have any bad luck and have just one bad day in the mountains, you can still finish in the top 10."

What about winning this Tour de France? It's a question usually asked by Americans who remember Greg LeMond's three victories and expected that now, with LeMond retired, Armstrong would step up and replace him on the victory podium.

"Hah," he snorted. "You get a few questions like that, certainly. I say I'd like to contend some day and I think I can. People are quick to categorize a guy, to say he can't climb the high mountains, he can't time-trial, he's too big, he can't recover." The first was often said then about Armstrong and the second sometimes.

"Well, you know, you can't say that. Certainly if my development curve continues to go in the way that it's been going, there's no reason that in five years I can't contend for this race.

"I'm not in any hurry. I'm not saying I have to do it this year. Which is nice."

Armstrong returned in June from the United States, where he won the Tour DuPont and the West Virginia Kmart Classic, to ride in the Tour of Switzerland, where he was fourth in the prologue and fifth in the uphill individual time-trial. Both were among his best results in similar European races.

"I feel a lot stronger than I did a year ago," he said. The reason, he explained, is "I'm another year older.

"I expect that progress. Just as I expect a year from I'll be stronger than I am now. I'm only 23 years old. I fully expect to have steps like that for the next five years. That's reasonable, that's natural and normal.

"Mentally, I'm much better than I was three or four months ago. More focused." Credit for that, he said, went to his "very satisfying" victory in the DuPont, in which he finished second the previous two years. Armstrong likes to win and he likes to win in the United States.

In the Tour, he said, the daily stages that offered him his best chances came during the second week, on the trek from the Alps to the Pyrenees. He flipped through cards showing the profiles of each day's course.

"I really like this day," he said of the 12th stage, from St. Etienne to Mende. "Look at that finish," a short, sharp climb. "I like this one too," the 13th stage, from Mende to Revel. "It'll be hot and I like that and all these ups and downs, I like that."

He turned over a few more cards, their jagged profiles showing the mountains to be labored up, the descents to be sped down.

"It looks pretty easy this year, the Tour de France," Armstrong decided.

He paused a beat, and smiled. "I don't think so," he said.

July 18, 1995
Death of a Friend

Crashing on a sinuous and steep descent in the Pyrenees, Fabio Casartelli, a 24-year-old Italian rider for the Motorola team, was killed in the Tour de France. It was only the third death of a rider since the race began in 1903.

Casartelli died of a fractured skull, apparently after his head hit one of the concrete blocks that line the roadway. He fell in a multiple crash on the descent after the first of the day's climbs in the toughest stage of the race.

Flown by helicopter to a hospital in Tarbes, Casartelli suffered three heart stoppages and was revived after the first two by doctors aboard the aircraft. They were unsuccessful after the third attack.

The fatality was the first in the Tour since 1967. Tom Simpson, a British rider, died in July of that year of heat asphyxiation, complicated by amphetamine use, while climbing Mont Ventoux.

Casartelli, who won a gold medal in the road race at the 1992 Olympics in Barcelona, would have been 25 the next month. He was married and had a 4-month-old son.

After he crashed on the descent from the Portet d'Aspet Pass, the first of six climbs that day in the Pyrenees, Dr. Gerard Porte, one of the Tour's four doctors, said he knew at once that the rider was critically injured.

"I arrived 10 seconds after the fall," he said. "I could tell it was a serious injury. Casartelli had cuts that were bleeding badly.

"We did everything in the best conditions and as fast as we could," the doctor said. "But he had very serious cuts, and when there's such heavy bleeding you know it was a very powerful impact."

Casartelli was not wearing a helmet, which is not mandatory except in the Benelux countries. Even there, helmets are often the strips of leather known as "hairnets," rather than more resistant hard-shell gear.

Despite the obvious dangers, few professional riders wear helmets on hot days, insisting that for comfort's sake they prefer cloth caps or bare heads. When international officials tried to make helmets mandatory early in the 1990s, the riders threatened to strike and the officials backed off.

Three other riders were injured in the crash. Dante Rezze, a Frenchman with the Aki team, went off the road and into a ravine, fracturing his left leg. Dirk Baldinger, a German with Polti, also fractured his left leg. Juan Cesar Aguirre, a Colombian with Kelme, was less seriously injured but still had to withdraw from the race. Rezze and Baldinger were both taken by ambulance to the town of St. Gaudens.

Dr. Gerard Nicolet, another of the Tour's doctors, and Dr. Massimo Testa, the Motorola team's doctor, accompanied Casartelli on the helicopter and tried to save him.

The accident occurred at Kilometer 34 of the 206-kilometer (128-mile) stage in sunny, hot weather.

July 19, 1995
Paying Homage

Stunned, saddened and in some cases demoralized, the 118 remaining riders in the Tour set off the next day on a selfless journey.

By common consent, from Miguel Indurain in the leader's yellow jersey to Hector Castano in last place, the daily stage was dedicated to the memory of Fabio Casartelli. Even though he had neglected to wear a helmet in the heavy heat of the day, just a handful of riders wore hard helmets the next day, including only Lance Armstrong and Alvaro Mejia, a Colombian, of the six remaining members of the nine-man Motorola squad.

Like probably 90 percent of the pack, the four other Motorola riders wore cloth caps or rode bareheaded. They also wore black patches pinned to their left sleeves. Applauded by a huge crowd of spectators before the start, most of the Motorola riders refused to comment and rode away to take their places in the front line of the pack for a minute of silence for their dead teammate.

"The team decided to stay in the race for the memory of Casartelli," Paul Sherwen, a Motorola spokesman, reported. "They felt it was easier to stay together as a group than to split up and go home each his separate way. Even if they didn't race today, they'd still have to race next week or the week after."

But this 16th of 20 stages in the Tour was not a race. It was a procession. The riders remained grouped throughout, traveling at the stately pace of 30 kilometers an hour (18.6 miles an hour), about 10 km/h below their average in the three-week race.

Shoulder to shoulder, rank after rank, they traveled the 237 kilometers from Tarbes to Pau over six climbs in the Pyrenees. Attacks were forbidden and riders who fell behind on the climbs were given time to catch up: The pack's leaders decreed beforehand that all riders show solidarity to the memory of Casartelli.

In the same spirit, Andrea Peron, a fellow Italian and Casartelli's roommate with Motorola, was allowed to win the stage. The same gesture was made in 1967, when Tom Simpson died up Mont Ventoux. The next day the pack allowed his teammate and countryman Barry Hoban to win in a long breakaway.

This time the rest of the pack let the remaining six Motorola riders move to the front with 10 kilometers to go. When one of the men, Stephen Swart of New Zealand, then had to stop because of a flat and have a wheel replaced, the entire pack slowed to await his return.

In the final few kilometers, the six — Frankie Andreu, Steve Bauer, Armstrong, Mejia, Swart, and Peron — rode alone as the rest of the pack dropped a few hundred meters back.

Abreast as the finish line approached, the Motorola riders coasted over together with Peron the first to cross in an immensely moving ceremony. All other placings, from second to 118th, were irrelevant. The pack was one man in this stage.

In addition to the tribute of victory for Peron, Motorola riders were allowed to win the stage's first sprint and first two climbs. All prizes for the day, amounting to 225,000 French francs (about $45,000), were donated to Casartelli's widow and were matched by the Tour's organizers.

The Motorola team also said it would donate all its prize money for the race, about 140,000 francs at that point, to the widow.

Casartelli's body was flown back to his village near Como for his funeral.

"Terrible, terrible for him and for us," said Gianluca Bortolami, an Italian with the Mapei team, before the start and its minute of silence for the dead rider. Bortolami said he had ridden on the same amateur team in Italy with Casartelli and last spoke with him two days before the fatal crash.

"He said how eager he was for the race to be over so he could see his wife and son," said Bortolami, who wore a black ribbon pinned to his team jersey on the right side of his chest. Casartelli's son was a few months old.

"Terrible for our morale," Bortolami continued. "It makes you wonder about the point of continuing to Paris."

Like most of the riders, Bortolami did not wear a hard helmet in this stage. Instead he was bareheaded in the heavy heat that enveloped Tarbes even in mid-morning.

"What's the point of wearing a helmet," he said. "If you wear it today," for symbolic purposes, "you won't wear it tomorrow."

July 21, 1995
One for Casartelli

In an emotional ride that he said was dedicated to and inspired by his dead teammate, Lance Armstrong won the 18th stage of the Tour de France, blowing a kiss to the heavens as he crossed the finish line.

"This was for Fabio Casartelli," Armstrong said. "I was very, very bad in the last bit, but I kept thinking of him. I did it for one person," the dead Italian rider.

Although the Tour's riders paid him tribute the day after his death by allowing the remaining six Motorola riders to pass over the finish line together and ahead of the pack, let no one imagine that this victory was handed to Armstrong. The Texan rode away from a 12-man breakaway and built his lead until he arrived in Limoges ahead by 33 seconds.

With one kilometer to go, Armstrong looked back and saw no opponents down the road. He pointed to the sky with his right hand, then both hands and finally blew a kiss upward.

"Everybody loved him," he said of Casartelli afterward. "He was a super person, he had more friends than anybody I've ever known."

Before the start, Armstrong seemed more animated than he had been since the fatal crash. "I'm starting to feel better about what happened," he said in a brief conversation as he signed autographs for fans and tried to weave through the crowd for a coffee. "It's natural, I'm beginning to put it in the past."

Before the Tour began in Brittany, the Texan said his goals included finishing the race for the first time, winning a stage and perhaps finishing in the top 15. Asked whether he wanted the top 15 ranking or the stage victory more, he replied, "The stage victory. There's no doubt there."

Now he had it and shortly he would finish the Tour for the first time. The last goal was beyond his reach: He ranked 36th, one hour 21 minutes 22 seconds behind the leader, Miguel Indurain.

"I'm no Miguel Indurain, no way," Armstrong said. "I think his engine is bigger than mine."

With only a couple of stages left, many riders tried to attack in what for most was their last chance at a victory in this Tour. They were all apprehended until, at Kilometer 83, six riders bolted off.

They were joined shortly by six more, including Armstrong. Since 10 of the race's 21 teams were represented in the breakaway, the chase after them was minimal.

The 12 were not allowed, however, to build a huge margin. On the last major climb, Armstrong caught his companions thinking of other matters and jumped away from them just before the peak. At that point, riders are often relaxed, believing that the worst of the climb is over and not expecting an attack. About 30 kilometers remained in the stage.

"I didn't like my chances in the sprint and I thought I'd better try to put them away early," he said. "I had a feeling that they couldn't put a chase together."

They couldn't. Working together raggedly, the chasers let Armstrong build his lead from a handful of seconds to a peak of 1:03 with five kilometers to go. The time came down on the final uphill two kilometers to the finish, but Armstrong had a clear road behind him.

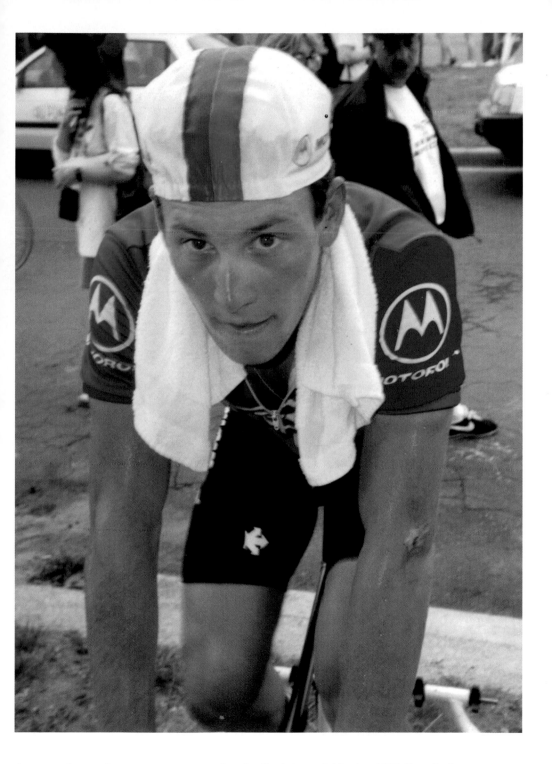

An eager Lance Armstrong warms up for the final time trial in the 1992 Tour DuPont.
Although he was already a member of the Motorola team, he was still racing as an amateur.

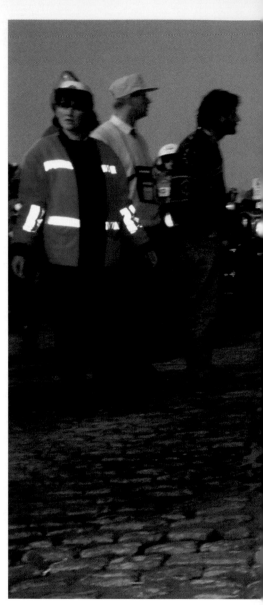

Below: Victory in Belgium's grueling Flèche Wallone race cemented Armstrong's reputation as a top classics rider.

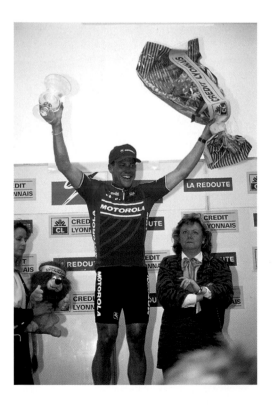

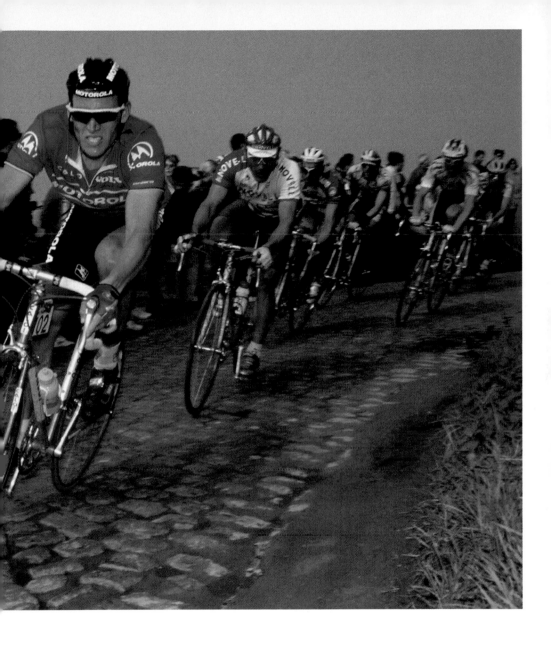

Above: In his early years as a professional, Armstrong focused on one-day classics. Here he rounds a cobbled corner in the 1995 Tour of Flanders.

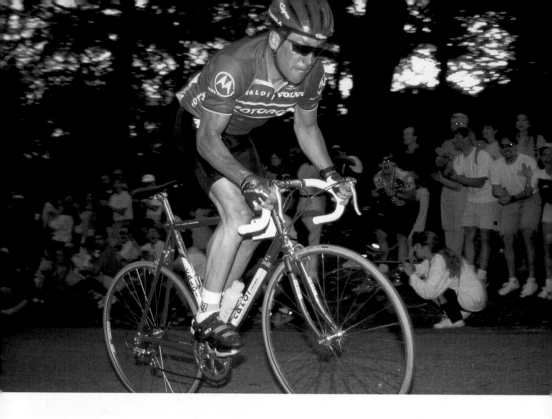

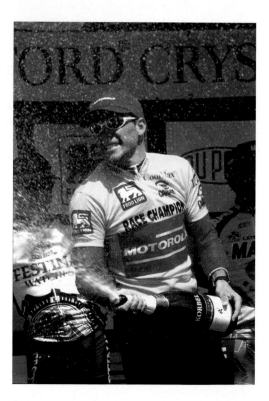

Above: Armstrong first gained respect as a stage racer by twice winning the Tour DuPont. Here he attacks on Taylor's Hill before rolling to victory in downtown Richmond, Virginia, during the 1996 event.

Left: With champagne and the yellow jersey, Lance Armstrong celebrates his second Tour DuPont victory in 1996.

Right: In a heart-rending press conference, the 23-year-old Armstrong tries to put his symbolic win into perspective. It would not be his last symbolic victory.

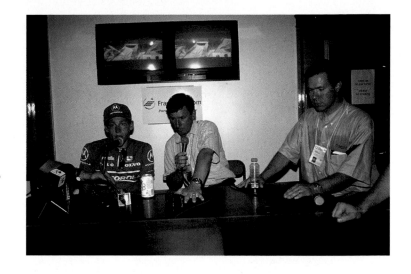

Below: The 1995 Tour de France was marked by the death of his Motorola teammate Fabio Casartelli. Three days later, Armstrong falls into the arms of his soigmeur after an emotional stage victory into Limoges.

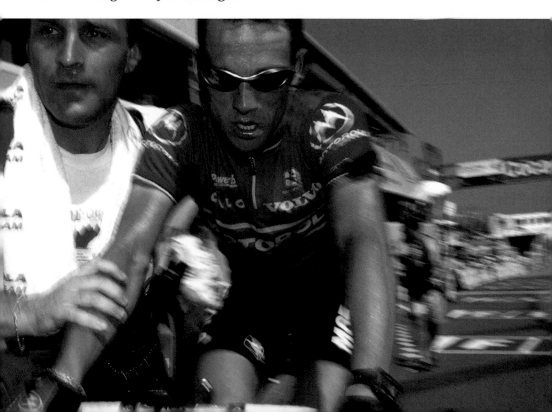

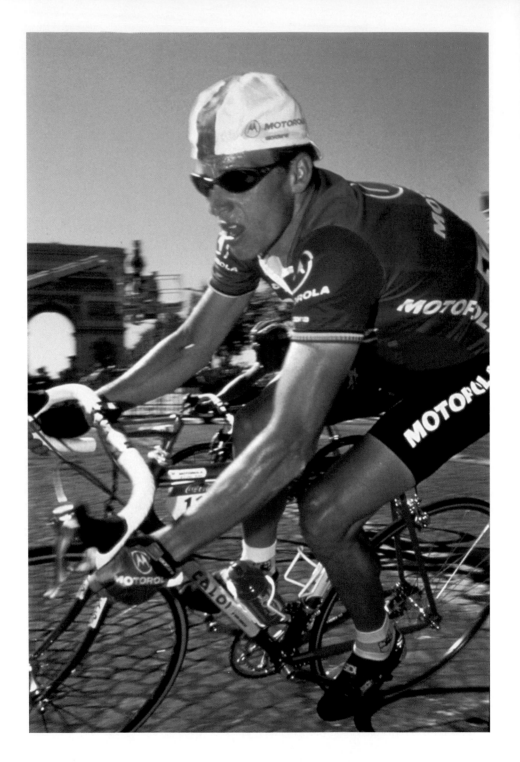

Only twice has Armstrong reached Paris at the conclusion of a Tour de France. Back in 1995, he finished 36th, 1 hour 28 minutes and 6 seconds behind Spain's Miguel Indurain.

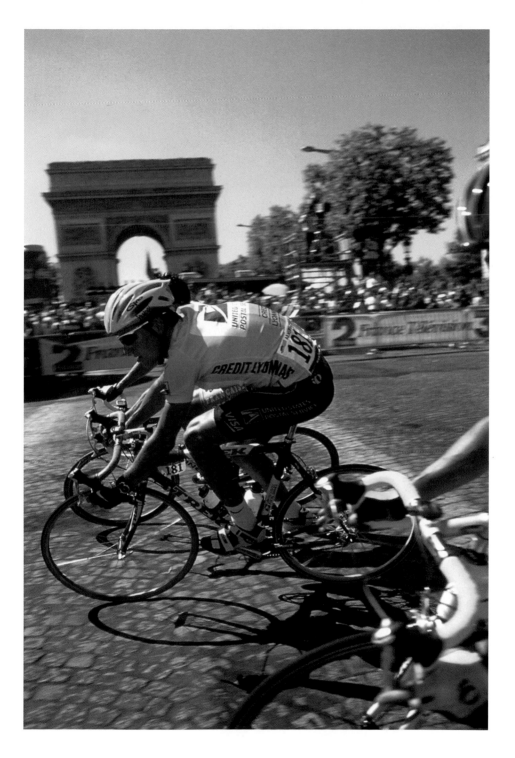

In 1999, after 91 hours 32 minutes and 16 seconds of racing, Armstrong finished behind no one, winning the Tour de France convincingly.

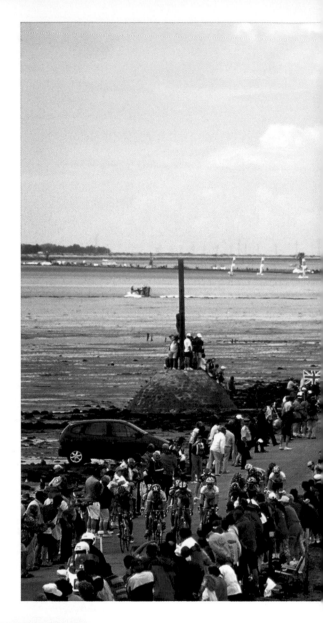

Below: Estonian sprinter Jaan Kirsipuu would be the only other rider in the 1999 Tour de France to wear the yellow jersey.

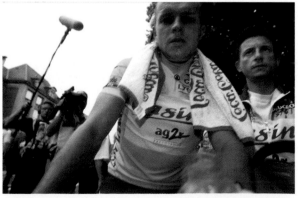

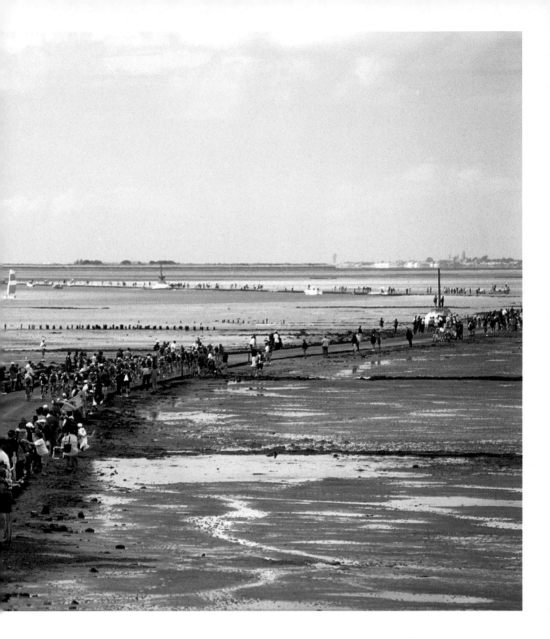

Above: His experience as a classics rider, as well as a the support of a strong team, helped Armstrong get across the treacherous Passage du Gois in the lead group during Stage 2 of the 1999 Tour, while rivals, such as Switzerland's Alex Zülle and Holland's Michael Boogerd lost over six minutes.

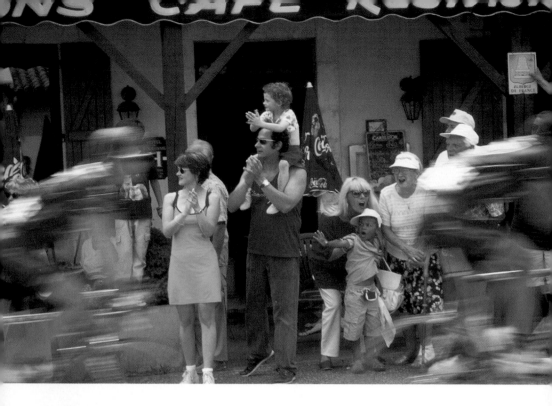

Above: The U.S. Postal Service team leads the charge through rural France on Stage 14 to Saint Gaudens. For nearly a century now, the Tour has attracted the country's imagination.

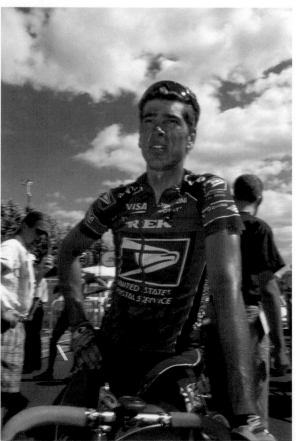

Left: Since 1992, Michigan native Frankie Andreu has ridden with Armstrong. And over the years he has proven to be the Texan's most faithful teammate.

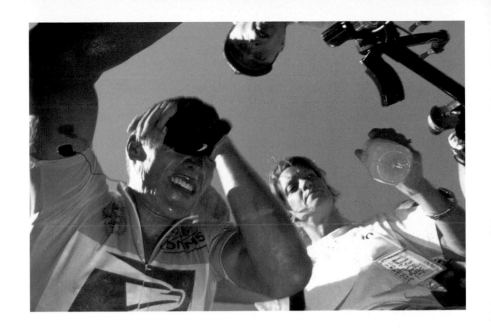

Above: Seconds after the final time trial in Futuroscope, things were difficult. Seemingly only the bike could keep the yellow jersey propped up.

Below: Cruising through a descent in the Pyrenees, Armstrong makes bike racing look easy...

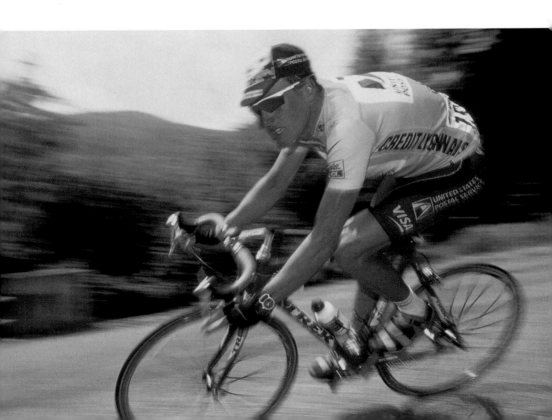

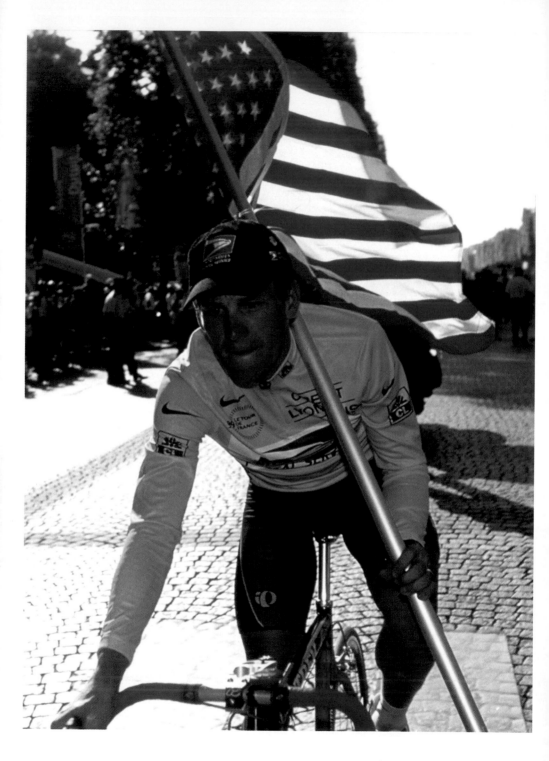

Always a proud American, Armstrong cruises down the Champs Élysées waving the stars and stripes after final victory in the 1999 Tour de France.

July 25, 1995
Homage to Big Mig

Pronouncing himself Miguel Indurain's biggest fan, Lance Armstrong had a small doubt before the Tour de France began that the Spaniard could win the bicycle race for a record fifth consecutive year.

"The numbers, I'm aware of the numbers," said Armstrong. "If I'm playing the numbers, it's never been done."

Now it had. Indurain, who rode for the Banesto team, joined Jacques Anquetil, Eddy Merckx and Bernard Hinault as the only riders ever to win the Tour five times. Since the race began in 1903, he was the only man to win it five years running.

That convinced Armstrong that numbers are overrated.

"He's won five in a row and I say he'll win seven in a row," the Texan said as he turned in his bicycle to mechanics after the finish. "He's great, he's super," Armstrong said with enthusiasm about his role model. "He's the biggest engine ever to hit the sport; he's one of the classiest guys out there. He's too good, too good.

"He's too professional, his team is too professional. He's got it down. I could be wrong, but I'm now saying seven in a row."

The American was in an expansive mood after the finish, having fulfilled two of his three goals: He finished and he won a daily stage, although he failed to reach the top 15, ending in 36th place. That was the lowest-rated goal anyway and so Armstrong was happy to be signing autographs, posing for pictures with fans, and accepting congratulations for his stage victory, for finishing the Tour for the first time in three rides and for dealing so admirably with the death of his teammate Fabio Casartelli.

Life is a learning experience, agreed, and the 23-year-old Armstrong said he had learned a lot during the last three weeks about professional bicycle racing and about life itself.

"In cycling, I learned what it's like to do a three-week race," he explained. "Hard, very hard. But the last few days I felt so good that I think I'm coming out of this race in a good way.

"The race did a lot for me in terms of riding three weeks. People say once you do a big Tour, then you're a different rider. It changes you. I don't exactly expect to be the strongest guy in the peloton now because I finished the Tour de France, but I do expect it to give me some strength. I'm certainly coming out of the race healthy."

An Italian fan tapped him and said, "Bravo."

"Grazie," Armstrong replied.

Then an American couple pushed up to him and the woman told him: "We're very proud of you (thank you). You represent us well (thank you)."

"People are nice," Armstrong said.

That brought him to the Casartelli death.

"Certainly I learned more about life and death in this Tour than I learned about bike racing," he said. "More than anything else I learned how to deal with death.

"I had to deal with the death of a teammate and that's something I never faced before. I never had to deal with the death of a family member, a friend, a teammate ever before. Ever.

"This is the first one. And to have it happen in the Tour de France, it was very difficult," he said.

He handled it well, a friend said, citing the way he pointed to the sky at the end of the stage victory that Armstrong said was inspired by and dedicated to Casartelli.

"I didn't," Armstrong began. "I didn't," he repeated. Then he found the words.

"That was a special day. Those weren't my legs. Because they were way too good. They were so good.

"The week before that I was physically so tired and the legs that day, they showed up, the breakaway showed up and that attack I made — in the last 25 kilometers to go 55 to 60 kilometers an hour on a false-flat uphill.

"Come on. I've never in my life ridden a bike that fast. Those were very special kilometers there.

"It's hard to explain, it's unexplainable. The feeling was…" A long pause.

"Boy, I was so strong."

August 14, 1995
Victory in a Classic

Going from last place to first in three years, Lance Armstrong won the Clasica San Sebastian, his first victory in a World Cup bicycle race. In his initial race as a professional, in San Sebastian in 1992, he finished 111th, dead last and 11 lonely minutes behind the rider in 110th place.

Revenge? "No, not so much," he replied by phone from his home in Italy. In fact, he said, he had not thought of his debut during the victory. "It's still a pretty strong memory," he explained, "but I only thought of that race afterward."

His thoughts were positive, he continued. "It was probably one of the best things I could have done, not simply pulling over, dropping out when I was so far behind. Finishing that race said a lot about my character to the team and to the other riders: that I was not a quitter. That I was in the sport to finish."

This time around, he was an easy winner in Spain, completing the 234 kilometers (143 miles) in 5 hours 31 minutes 17 seconds, or 2 seconds faster in the final sprint than Stefano Della Santa, an Italian with the Mapei team.

In a sprint the year before in the same race, Armstrong beat Della Santa for second place. That was one of three second places he had recorded in World Cup races.

"I thought it was going to be second place again," Armstrong said. "That's what I was thinking about, not '92."

Until the last six kilometers, he was in a two-man breakaway with Laurent Jalabert, a Frenchman with ONCE and a faster sprinter than Armstrong. Behind them was a chase group including Johan Museeuw, a Belgian with Mapei and the leader of the World Cup. Museeuw's goal was to catch Jalabert, one of his main rivals in the standings.

"It was better for me when we all came together," he said. "That gave me a chance, which I figured I didn't have alone with Jalabert."

Soon after the two were caught, Della Santa jumped off and Armstrong immediately went after him. As he more or less expected, Jalabert and Museeuw remained behind, watching each other.

"It's a couple of years now I've been playing this World Cup game," the Texan said. "I've learned what to expect."

The two attackers opened a 25-second lead that held up despite Armstrong's frequent glances back for signs of chase. "You never know, man — there was serious horsepower behind us," he said. "Jalabert, Museeuw, they can dial it up. There's nothing worse than getting surprised from behind."

But in the straightaway to the finish, he and Della Santa were alone. Armstrong pulled left around his opponent and won easily. Museeuw was third, Jalabert fourth.

"Now I can approach the world championships with a clear mind," Armstrong concluded. "I don't need a victory there to save my season. It's not necessarily do or die."

March 13, 1996
An Uncertain Beginning

Usually so upbeat and optimistic, Lance Armstrong was sounding downcast and uncertain. With some of his most important races only weeks away in the new season, he could not tell how strong he was.

"Top form," he repeated. "I don't know about top form."

The problem was a bad crash in the Tour of Valencia in Spain at the start of the month. Armstrong was on a rapid descent and possibly heading for victory when he skidded on gravel and fell. He needed a week off to recover, and a week was a long time for a rider to be away from his bicycle this early in the season.

"I'm in good form," Armstrong admitted. "I have to see how I recovered from this crash. I certainly was heading in the right direction, but it's difficult to say now. A week off."

"I'll find out today how much of an effect it had on me," he said as he awaited the start of the third stage of the Paris–Nice race. "Today's hard," he continued. "There are gonna be people everywhere today."

How right he was. The 151 riders arrived scattered at the end of the 170.5-kilometer (106-mile) stage from Vassivière-en-Limousin to the village of Chalvignac. The easy winner, by 16 seconds, was Laurent Jalabert, the top-ranked rider in the world.

"No doubt about it," Armstrong said, "the best man won."

He had the credentials to judge, since he finished second — and did not seem reassured.

"I still don't feel the way I did a week ago," Armstrong said as he toweled his face and arms. "I just don't have the punch. That was the difference. Jalabert's strong. He's a sprinter, so he has a lot of acceleration."

Shoulder to shoulder with the American, Jalabert pulled ahead halfway up the 3.8-kilometer steep climb to the finish line and kept opening the gap.

Although Armstrong beat Chris Boardman in the sprint for second, he was not satisfied afterward.

"I definitely wasn't good enough today to win a classic," he said.

Since that was his main objective in the World Cup series, the timing of his crash could not have been worse. The Milan–San Remo race opened the World Cup late in March and was followed on April weekends by the Tour of Flanders, Paris–Roubaix, Liège–Bastogne–Liège and the Amstel Gold Race.

All except Paris–Roubaix ranked among the Texan's favorite races, especially Liège, where he had finished second and sixth in the last two years.

Looking ahead, Armstrong continued in his gloomy mode. Of Milan–San Remo, for example, he said: "I think that race suits my characteristics, but I always seem to have a bad day there. In the last two years I've gone in with high hopes and was disappointed. But I still think it's a good race for me." He was 73rd the year before.

"Flanders is another big objective," he continued. "Again a race that I think suits me, although I've always had a bad day there. I think it's time I had a good day." He was 45th the year before.

"I have to see what happens here," he said, referring to Paris–Nice. He won a stage in the race the year before and, off his form before the crash in Spain, was considered to be an outside favorite.

In many ways, a one-week race like Paris–Nice should have been ideal for his ambitions then. He said he had worked hard at home in Austin to prepare for the spring races. "I did a hard winter," he reported with a certain pride. "I started earlier than usual, close to the beginning of November. But not seriously riding a bike. I did some weight training, which I'd never done before, not consistently.

"Lifting weights, I think that helped. I have more power, I'm stronger than other years. It was from the waist down, all leg training. I did no upper body stuff," which builds useless muscle mass for a bicycle racer.

"I did an awful lot of work to have a crash set me back," he said unhappily.

May 13, 1996
Downsized

Like any victim of corporate downsizing, Lance Armstrong seemed subdued and thoughtful as he examined his options after the Motorola electronics company announced that it would withdraw at the end of the 1996 season as a sponsor of the bicycle team he led.

The search was on for a new sponsor, preferably a multinational company based in the United States, willing to put up about $5 million a year into one of the sport's strongest teams.

Even though Armstrong did not have a guaranteed job for the next season, he knew that at 24 and as a racer approaching his peak, he would not have to start selling insurance on commission. The phone from prospective employers would start ringing shortly at his new home in Austin, where he planned to spend the next few weeks. In fact, he admitted, although he preferred to stay with the teammates and organization wearing Motorola's blue and red, he had already had some preliminary contacts with European teams.

"I started in April talking with teams." he said. "I'm not saying who. Just feeling it out a little bit. Even if Motorola announced today they would do two more years, I don't have a contract beyond this season.

"So it's normal to talk to other teams," he continued. "I have to figure out my value. But how much time do I have? I don't know. Good question. Space on teams goes fast.

"And money. That kind of money is not easy to come by. That's the reason I started in April. It's never too early."

He was making at least $750,000 that season and should have been eligible for a raise based on his superlative spring, including second place in Paris–Nice and Liège–Bastogne–Liège and victory in the Flèche Wallonne and the Tour DuPont. He ranked seventh in the ranking of the world's hundreds of professional riders.

Those results from somebody who said he despised the cold and rainy weather of spring races were no fluke. "This winter I was extremely motivated," he explained, "because I knew my contract was finished this year. I had a feeling Motorola wouldn't return. So, for 1997, to have to go out and maybe find a new team, find a new contract, find a new salary, I had to be super."

71

He said also that he had been changed by the death of Fabio Casartelli in the previous Tour de France: "It did change me, it did. It changed everybody in the Motorola program and I think it changed everybody in the sport to an extent.

"Now I realize that not only my career and my contract are precious but your life is precious. At the same time that I was worried about not having a contract next year, he doesn't have a life any more."

Although rumors said that Motorola would drop out as a sponsor after six years, a long stay in the sport, the formal announcement that spring came when the team was making its biggest impact. Armstrong and his teammates had never ridden more strongly, dominating some spring classics in Europe and especially the 12-day, 1,225-mile (1,960-kilometer) Tour DuPont, which Armstrong won.

"Obviously, results didn't factor into their decision," he said.

What would Armstrong say about himself if, in his job search, he had to run a classified ad? "You mean like white single male seeks white single female?

"OK, this is what I would say: I can be competitive in classic races, hard classic races," meaning one-day races. "I can be competitive in 7-to-10-day stage races. I can't guarantee you that I can win the Tour de France, I can't guarantee you that I can win field sprints, I can't guarantee you that I can win the climb to Alpe d'Huez, but I can certainly be a contender."

If Jim Ochowicz, the team's general manager, did not find a new sponsor by the Tour de France in July, Armstrong planned to sign with another team: "If he tells me he thinks something's going to come through, then I can wait. Because I trust him. But if he comes to me and says I really can't find anything, which he would do, he would tell me, then I would go away immediately."

He would not sign with a team based primarily in the United States: "I have goals in this sport that I want to achieve and I could go with Saturn or Postal Service, an American team, but I would not achieve my goals with them. I realize I have to go somewhere European if this team doesn't continue.

"I just hope it continues, I really do. It would be a shame if it didn't. The thing I'm most scared about is that this would have to end, that there wouldn't be a big-time American presence in Europe, in the classics, in the Tour de France.

"The sport needs that and I think American cycling needs that. That's my biggest concern."

July 5, 1996
Dreaming of Other Roads

Along with the other riders in the Tour de France, Lance Armstrong rode languidly south, heading toward the Alps and a long weekend of climbing.

Down Departmental Route 33 from the start in the Lac de Madine park they came, along Route 164 in the Vosges region, finishing the 242-kilometer (150-mile) fifth stage into the city of Besançon on twisty and narrow Route 70.

In heavy headwinds and frequent drenching rain, Armstrong was concentrating on those roads, of course, but part of his mind was on another thoroughfare: Peachtree Street in Atlanta. That would be the hub of the bicycle road race in the 1996 Olympic Games.

The Texan was focused on that 221.8-kilometer race, Scheduled 10 days after the Tour ended. "Obviously that's what makes the most sense for me as a goal," he said, referring to the Games, in which he was also scheduled to ride in the time-trial. "They're in America and they're the Olympics — the combination is big. I'm looking forward to them, yes I am."

The Games in Atlanta were the first open to professional riders, many of whom competed in the Olympics before as amateurs. Armstrong did, in Barcelona in 1992, and right afterward he turned professional and now ranked fourth in the world on one computerized list of racers.

But he was not shining in the overall standings in the 83rd Tour, resting in 54th place, 5 minutes 3 seconds behind. "Now is my time to lay low and prepare," he said. "In Atlanta and the World Cup races in August, the spotlight will be on me, but it isn't right now."

However, he intended to do his preparatory work in the Tour. While he did not intend to ride for a high place in the overall standings — "no, no, no, absolutely not," he said — Armstrong had definite objectives in the 3,900-kilometer race.

"I'll ride all the time-trials 100 percent," he said, "not go very deep in the mountains and try to select stages to do something, mainly in the second half."

He did not feel under any pressure, he continued, to prove anything in the Tour for a prospective new employer before the season ended and Motorola dropped its sponsorship. "If what I've done doesn't impress a sponsor, what can I do next?" he asked. "I think we've got a very good Tour team, and I'll do all I can to help my teammates.

"It's fair to say I'm looking ahead to the Olympics, but certainly I recognize the importance of the Tour de France, its magnitude," Armstrong continued. "I'm not here to be just trying, I'm not here on vacation. I'm ready."

His physical condition, he reported, was "probably about 75 percent." After his easy DuPont victory that May, he went back to Austin, moved into his new home, and took a month off. "Mentally that was good for me," he said, "physically I probably relaxed a little too much."

Armstrong was familiar with the Olympic route. "It's not the best course for me," he said. "It's just not challenging, not super- challenging." The course was flat, with one small climb.

"I don't think the course will be very selective," Armstrong said, meaning that weaker riders would not be weeded out early. "It'll be more random and tactical — which is unfortunate in such a big event, but they're not going to change it. I'll have to do what I can. The good thing about the course is that it's right in town and there should be a lot of people there, a lot of support, I hope."

July 6, 1996
Cold, Wet, and Sick

As thunder roared and rain pelted down for another day, Lance Armstrong decided that an overnight sickness had robbed him of his power and that he could not continue in the Tour de France.

"I couldn't breathe," he said after his withdrawal. "I started feeling a little sick last night. I'm never sick, and I didn't tell anyone I was sick.

"I'm bummed," he said, looking weary and depressed, nowhere near his usual ebullient self. "If I'm sick, I'm sick, and I have to stop."

The first hour of the stage, he continued, "was easy. Then it started going hard and I had no power. I couldn't breathe."

Armstrong fell behind the pack just before the second of five climbs over hills in the Jura and Savoy regions in eastern France. The sixth stage lasted 207 kilometers (128 miles) from Arc-et-Senans to the lakeside resort of Aix-les-Bains, usually in sight of the Alps. But not this day, not with the curtains of rain whipped by heavy wind.

Once he dropped back, Armstrong raised a hand to signal for his Motorola team car. When it arrived, Jim Ochowicz asked him if he wanted teammates to drop back and help tow him to the pack. The rider said he declined because he knew he could not make it to the finish even with help.

He struggled on alone for about 20 kilometers before he coasted to the side of the road and stopped. An official removed the number 61 pinned on the back of his shorts and Armstrong was officially out of the race.

He then remounted his bicycle, turned, and rode back down the road, away from the other riders, knowing that another team car was far back and that he could get a ride in it to the team's hotel.

This was the third time in his four Tours de France that he has not made it to the finish, although the first two withdrawals were programmed because of his age and inexperience.

He was not the only man to drop out — 12 other riders also did. Weeklong rains and strong wind had forced the riders to strain in high gears, producing an epidemic of knee injuries, and the slick roads had caused many crashes.

Armstrong was the Motorola team's most visible member, and his loss would probably be a blow to the efforts of Ochowicz to find another American sponsor. Ochowicz said that he remained hopeful, but still had no word from what he described as "the three or four companies that are interested." The clock was ticking.

"As of today, we have no one signed on," he said. "Our absolute drop-dead date is September 1. That's a signed, sealed, and delivered contract.

"We could get a commitment during the Tour, and it could take 30 or 45 days to get the contract done, but we can go forward if we get a letter of commitment."

August 29, 1996
No Sign of the Cavalry

The last-minute rescue almost certainly would not occur, Lance Armstrong realized. The cavalry would not be coming over the hill. Weeks past what was once a firm deadline to find a new sponsor, the Motorola team still was looking for a company to enable it to continue in the next season.

Armstrong was willing to wait a bit longer. He remained hopeful, he said over the phone from the Netherlands, where he was riding in the Tour of Holland.

"I don't know why it shouldn't happen," he said, referring to a reprieve. But, he admitted, he had been saying that for months. Jim Ochowicz had spoken to many potential sponsors and come up empty.

"Och has had four or five people who have led him along, led him along, told him they're definitely going to do his bike team, and then the bottom falls out," Armstrong said bitterly. September is usually the month that riders announce that they are moving to a new team, and Armstrong thought that if he had such news to make public, he would do it then. He was not yet prepared to make that announcement although, he confirmed, he had made a verbal commitment to a new team if Ochowicz could not find the money to continue.

"I've signed nothing," the Texan said. "But I've narrowed my choices down to one if Jim is ultimately out, which I think he is."

While Armstrong would not say which team that was, it was the new Cofidis team, based in France. Negotiations with the Festina team, also based in France, fell through in July. "They were interested, but they didn't want to give me the time. They wanted a decision in July, and I wasn't prepared to make a decision in July."

After he dropped out of the Tour de France because of illness and returned home to Texas, Armstrong was notified by fax of Festina's lack of further interest. "That says a lot about the organization," he said. "That's OK. They'll realize soon enough."

The experience taught him that a deal is not final until the papers are signed. So, for now, he was officially refusing comment about which jersey he would be wearing when the next season opened.

He had been riding well that fall after an impressive spring. "It's the best season I've ever had," he decided. "I'm ecstatic about my season. My number one goal was to have a fantastic spring, and in the middle of May, I was the number one rider in the world."

Beginning in July, however, he declined. First he had to quit the Tour de France because he became ill and thought that riding in the constant rain would impede his chances in the Olympic Games. Then in Atlanta, he rode honorably if not overwhelmingly. "It was difficult to not have done the Tour and just to have trained," he said of his preparation for the Olympics. He finished 14th in the road race and sixth in the time-trial. "Of course I would have liked to have done better," he said, "but it's bike racing. Sometimes it works, sometimes it doesn't."

In the previous few weeks he had been 14th in the Clasica San Sebastian, fourth in the Leeds International Classic and fourth again in the Grand Prix of Zurich. Overall, he ranked 10th in the world and fifth in the standings of the World Cup. Although victory in the World Cup was one of his goals at the start of the season, he planned to drop out of competition by mid-September, returning home before the season wound up at the end of October. "It's not realistic to think you can go from March to November," he said. "I just want to spend some time at home."

His off-season activities, he added, would include language lessons if he moved to another team. "I'm prepared," he said. "I'll spend the entire winter tutoring. I don't want to go to a foreign team and be a foreigner. If you're the leader, you have to be able to communicate. I've been in this team five years and seen guys come and go who won't learn English. It just doesn't work. A leader whose teammates see him not even making an effort, you shoot yourself right in the foot."

September 3, 1996
Making It Official

The new Cofidis team announced that Lance Armstrong would be its leader next season. The team was expected to be directed by Cyrille Guimard of France — the man who launched the careers of Bernard Hinault, Laurent Fignon, and Greg LeMond.

Armstrong had signed a two-year contract that was believed to be for $1.25 million a year, part of which he was quietly refunding to the sponsor to help it hire Frankie Andreu, his American teammate and friend from Motorola.

Part III.
Down but Fighting Back

October 8, 1996
Terrible News

Lance Armstrong revealed from his home in Texas that he had testicular cancer, that it had spread to his abdomen and lungs, and that he had just started 12 weeks of chemotherapy.

"I intend to beat this disease," he said in an international conference call. "It's impossible to say when I'll be back racing, but I hold out hope to participate at the professional level in the 1997 season."

He noted that the survival rate from testicular cancer was 97 percent but that, "if it spreads, which it has, that number comes down."

He said his doctor put his chances of recovery between 65 and 85 percent and described the state of his abdominal cancer as "between moderate and advanced."

"I had four hours of chemotherapy yesterday," Armstrong said, "and if I didn't know the diagnosis, I'd feel normal."

Discussing his illness, Armstrong said, "It happened very fast." Not a week before, he felt severe pain in a testicle, coughed up blood and went to see Dr. Dudley Youman at St. David's Hospital in Austin. After an ultrasound examination, he was told of the cancer and the need to remove the testicle, which was done the next day.

At first, he said, he was incredulous. "I'm 25 years old," he related, "I'm one of the best in my sport — why would I have cancer? I had lots of tests all through my career, physical tests, blood tests, and they never picked this up.

"This is something I got stuck with and now have to work through," he continued. "I've said all along that I won't live as long as most people, this sport is too hard. The Tour de France is not a human event.

"But I'm entering this battle in the best shape of my life. I'm going to be back on my bike soon, maybe not six hours a day, maybe not as hard as before."

He said later that his doctor had approved bicycle riding up to 50 miles a day as early as the next week.

"I just want to be on my bike, outside, with my friends," Armstrong said. Throughout the hour-long conference call, he sounded buoyant and determined — two qualities, in addition to his talent, that have helped carry him to the top of his sport.

Although he had dropped out of the Tour de France that year in the first week, complaining that he had lost his power in cold and rainy weather and could not finish a daily stage, he now discounted chances that his cancer might have affected him then, noting that he rode well at the Olympic Games — 14th in the road race, 6th in the time-trial — and then in Europe that September, including fourth place in the Grand Prix of Switzerland.

He had finished his season in Europe that month by placing second in the Tour of Holland and finishing among the top five in two time-trials. "A month ago, I was in Europe competing at the highest level," he said in a wistful voice.

Only a month ago, he had signed a contract with Codifis. Officials of the French team said they were stunned to learn of Armstrong's illness a few days ago and cared now only about his recovery. He said he did not think he would lose his salary, adding that that was something to be worked out in the coming months.

"I've got bigger things to worry about," he said.

"This thing ain't going to stop me. I might have a bald head, but I'll be out there soon on my bike."

November 18, 1996
An Ordinary Morning

As mornings go, this one seemed ordinary: fog masked the hills west of Austin, a light wind fluttered flags, the temperature promised another shirt-sleeves day. About 7:30 o'clock, rain began falling for half an hour and everybody said that was a good thing because lately there had been a bit of a drought in central Texas.

A commonplace morning for most people, in other words, but another wonderful, joyful morning for Lance Armstrong. He woke at 7 at his home on Lake Austin, went to the kitchen to prepare a pink grapefruit for breakfast, looked at the morning newspaper and then began celebrating another day of simply being alive.

"Every day I wake up, I feel great," he said later. "I say 'This is great,' because six months from now, a year from now, five years from now, I may not be able to say that."

Two months before, Armstrong was competing and finishing high in long and arduous races in Europe. Then he was told that he had testicular cancer and that the cancer was also in his abdomen and lungs. Three weeks later, after the malignant testicle had been removed, he learned that the cancer had spread to his brain, requiring surgery to take out two lesions.

"You can see where they did it," he said. Lifting his blue Dallas Cowboys cap, he leaned forward to show the two stitched semicircles on the top left and back of his head. Somewhat proudly, he also showed two tiny bumps on either side of his forehead, where screws had held his head steady during the five-hour operation.

"I'm feeling fine," he said. "A little bit of fatigue, which means I have to take a nap every day, about two hours. This week I feel like I felt two months ago. I really do. That's no lie."

He was scheduled to leave in a couple of days for a week at the Indiana University Medical Center in Indianapolis, where he would receive four hours of chemotherapy daily for his third week. The treatment would be administered through a catheter that was surgically implanted and that he wore at home during the two weeks between each of four weeks of chemotherapy. Taped over his heart, the outside of the device resembled, ironically, the tube that bicycle riders use to pump air into flat tires.

He had no interest in irony, though. He was concentrating on one thing only and that was survival. For him, another morning alive was a triumph.

"It used to be when I woke up every morning, I knew I was going to wake up," he said. "It was so normal I took it for granted and now I never know. We're not promised anything. We're not promised tomorrow.

"We all expect to have long and fulfilling lives, but I suggest people not take that for granted. We don't always attack life, not do things to the fullest, and I suggest that people take advantage of life," he said.

He was sitting in the living room of his new, white Mediterranean-style villa, which he helped design. Circled by palm trees and clumps of flowers, the two-story house is airy and bright with high ceilings, vivid abstract painting and stylish furniture that he chose with his decorator. This is the house that he had dreamed about for years, perhaps as long ago as when he was a teenager living in Plano, outside Dallas, and growing up, as he describes it, "OK, middle class," raised by his mother, a single parent.

"This house, it represented a lot," he said in his living room. He had started talking outside, sitting near his swimming pool and hot tub, with a view across Lake Austin. It is also called the Colorado River, he explained, is 20 miles long from a spillway at one end to a dam at the other, and offers fine bass fishing. The view was splendid but the wind that moved the American and Texan flags on his shorefront was too cold for him, and he had to go inside.

A few months before, soon after he moved in, he said, "I'm happier here than I expected to be, and I expected to be very happy. Now that he had cancer, his feelings about his new house were more mixed.

"The home, I put a lot into it both in time and money, and I really feel an attachment to this house because this was dirt before, this was level ground and we built it up, furnished it, did everything exactly the way I wanted it. When I started it, I must have been 22 and it showed that a 22-year-old can work hard, financially do well and take on a big project like this and succeed. I've enjoyed it, I enjoy it still. But if it's gone, it's gone.

"Now it means a lot less than it did before. Houses, cars, motorcycles, toys, money, fame — it takes on a whole new meaning when you have something like this," he continued, referring to his cancer. "You realize, 'I never lived for that stuff.' No. I enjoyed it, but I think something like this makes you not only look at your life, but makes you simplify your life. The home means more than the other things. Before, I would have been devastated if I had to sell it or move out to a little old home built in the '30s, much smaller, not on the lake, not in this price range. That's fine. I could do it. That's fine, I'm alive. That's what it's all about."

The tan that he wears during the racing season had disappeared and he seemed pale, understandably less buoyant than usual. He was holding his weight steady at 170 pounds, he said, although he admitted that some of his muscle has turned to fat despite daily bicycle rides of up to an hour and a half.

"I do feel good," he said. "I'm not as fit as I used to be, but, then again, for two months I haven't done much on the bike. I'm undergoing chemotherapy and I do have cancer, pulmonary lesions that are detrimental. But the lesions on the lungs are going away pretty rapidly.

"I'm really upbeat. I'm positive. I may be a little scared, I may be very scared, but I feel very positive about how things are going."

A week earlier he even competed, with the legendary Eddy Merckx as his partner, in a local 26-mile race, the Tour of Gruene, Texas. "It was a race," he said, "but we didn't race. I can't race right now. I don't known if I can ever race again.

"I wanted to do the race to prove that I was still alive, that I was well, that therapy was ahead of schedule, as well as to prove to cancer patients that cancer doesn't always have to be a killer, therapy doesn't always have to be such a handicap."

Armstrong said that measurements of the level of proteins in his blood produced by the testicular cancer had gone from a high point of above 100,000 down to 113. "Still a way to go," he said. "That encourages me, even though the hardest part to knock out is the last part."

Those who knew Armstrong best agreed that he was doing well, physically and mentally. "He has met every benchmark of progress, and there's nothing to keep us from thinking he won't be cured," said

Dr. Craig Nichols on the phone from Indianapolis. He and Dr. Law-rence Einhorn were treating Armstrong at the Indiana University center.

"Lance's doing great," said Bill Stapleton, his agent, in Austin. "He's so upbeat, so confident," said Kevin Livingston, a teammate of Armstrong's with Motorola, who had moved to Austin to train with him, and then followed him to Cofidis.

"He's doing magnificently," said Armstrong's mother, Linda, on the phone from Richardson, Texas. "It's only a bump in the road. We're going to beat it. I tell him, 'Negatives don't do anything for you but bring you down,' and he knows that. 'Make this the first day of the rest of your life,' I say to him, and that's what he's doing."

Yes, he agreed, that was what he was doing.

"This is the biggest challenge of my life," he said. "Everything I've ever done has always been up to me. If I want to win a bike race, it's my responsibility to train hard, to eat right, to race smart — all things I could control. But now, I'd like to think that I can control things, but I don't know, I can only approach them in a way that I feel is appropriate — to fight with my mind and my body and just hope that things work out. I won't make you any guarantees in this fight.

"From the first moment I learned this, I thought, 'Oh my God, I'm going to die. I went from being at the top of my game, fourth in World Cup races in Leeds and Zurich, to being told I had cancer. Eventually you get over that. I said, 'Forget the numbers, forget the chances the doctors give you, forget it. We're going to work hard and we're going to win this. I'm not going to die, I'm going to live.' I chose to live, to fight to live.

"But if you're the biggest, toughest guy out there and saying, 'I'm going to live,' there are cases where you do die. Because cancer does not recognize that. It does not play fair. It's aggressive, it's smart, it's tough, it's relentless, it adapts, it becomes resistant to therapies. If it wants to win, it can win."

For now, he continued, he was giving little thought to his career as a bicycle racer.

Getting up from his chair to fetch another half grapefruit — "citrus fruits," he said, "they definitely fight cancer." He barely looked at a prospectus for the next Tour de France that a friend had brought him. "I think very little about that, maybe a quarter of the time," Armstrong said. "The other three quarters are focused on my life and beating cancer. If, for some reason, I can never race again, listen, that's fine."

The 1997 tour would be extremely mountainous and, he was told jokingly, would be a terrible tour for him. "Cancer is a terrible tour for me," he responded. "The Tour de France, it doesn't matter.

"I would love to race but nothing's going to make me happier than to live. Life is the number one priority. Professional cycling is number two. No, to create awareness for testicular cancer is number two. Professional cycling is number three.

"I would like to create a foundation for awareness of testicular cancer. I'd rather not have it but I've learned a lot about myself, about others and about life that most people never learn."

Did he feel that it was unjust that he had cancer? "No, because cancer doesn't play like that," he answered. "It doesn't play fair — nobody wants cancer. You can say, 'Why me?' but why not me? It doesn't strike because you've done something or not done something. I was just one of the ones it happened to hit.

"No, I don't want to waste my time saying, 'Why me?' I have a problem, and I want to fix it."

December 20, 1996
Good News

His doctors were optimistic, Lance Armstrong said, declaring after 12 weeks of chemotherapy and rest that he was in "partial remission" from cancer and that he did not need to see them again until a checkup in February. "I feel good, I don't feel sick, and I really do miss racing."

He had completed his scheduled treatment in Indianapolis the week before. "My blood level is normal now," Armstrong said on the phone from Austin. "The X-rays and CAT scan are not normalized yet, but that's because of the scar tissue. It takes time for the spots on my lungs and a spot on the abdomen to go away. But the doctors are optimistic. They say that my X-rays are exactly in line with a cure. They think this thing can be over."

So, he continued, it was back to work, however slowly. "I'll do the holidays first, and then it's back on my bike." Just after Christmas he planned to head to the heat and the flat roads of Miami to begin riding for longer spells than the occasional hour he had been logging in Austin's hills. "I'll go out as long as it's comfortable." he said.

His goal was to complete a four-hour ride before he came to France for the official presentation of his new team in January.

Beyond that, he admitted, his goals for the coming season were vague — his racing goals at any rate. "If you ask me what I hope for next year," he said, "it's just to keep living.

"I really have no idea when I might be back in a real race," he continued, "but I'm not going to be rushing it. I don't want to race until I'm ready physically. Mentally, my motivation is there. I really miss racing."

He was unsure how factors like motivation and desire would figure in his comeback. The physical demands of the sport — the eight-hour races over 250 kilometers (155 miles), often in the rain and cold of winter or the blazing heat of summer — might be overpowering.

Although he was hired to be Cofidis's leader, once his cancer was diagnosed, the team hired the Swiss star Tony Rominger as its leader. If Armstrong did not regain his full power and endurance, would he be comfortable as a support rider rather than a leader? "I would give it considerable time to see how far back I can come," he replied. He was unable to define how long would be considerable.

"But if I find out that I'm not real close to where I was before, I would move on," he decided. "There are a lot of other things to do with my life if I can't do racing."

January 15, 1997
From 90,000 to 3

His numbers were good and getting better, and so was he, Lance Armstrong said happily.

By "numbers," he meant his markers — the protein count in his blood that signified how his battle against cancer was progressing. "They're down to three," he said. "Three from a high of 90,000." Zero means the body is free of cancer.

His "numbers" also meant the odds that he would live and overcome the spread of testicular cancer after 12 weeks of chemotherapy. "At the end of the last treatment, I asked my doctor, 'If I was 50-50 before, where am I now?' He said 80-20. And that's a month ago."

Despite the improvement, Armstrong made no secret of his feelings. "It's scary," he said. "The longer I'm away from my exams, the more I get worried till I see the doctor again. It's such a relief when he says, 'You're getting well.'"

His next visit to his doctor in Indianapolis was scheduled in February. Armstrong, who was in Paris for the formal presentation of the Cofidis team, planned to fly home in a few days after spending nearly a week in France, meeting his new teammates, renegotiating his contract and resuming serious training. Until he began riding hard again in Florida late in December, he had not been training since he ended his season the September before.

"On the bike, I've never had to suffer as I did in the last few weeks," Armstrong said. "I tried to ride through the chemotherapy, but I had to ride slow and to go just that speed would hurt. That was a big adjustment. And off the bike, of course, there were many, many, many adjustments to make, just mentally, knowing you were fighting for your life."

His new team included three other American veterans of the extinct Motorola squad: Kevin Livingston, Bobby Julich, and Frankie Andreu. They said that Armstrong seemed fit enough, everything considered. "We rode about 120 kilometers yesterday," he reported. "I enjoy riding. Now it's physically easier. I feel stronger. Stronger, not strong."

When he returned to Texas, he planned to concentrate on weight training. "I'm going to start Monday as if I were starting in November or December, go back and do your typical off-season training, strength-building," he said. "Then I'll work on the aerobic engine." While he remained in Texas, the 20 other Cofidis riders would be starting their season — first with a training camp in the south of France, and then in races in February.

When the riders trooped on stage one by one at the team presentation, the Texan won the loudest ovation. His illness and recovery had been major news in Europe, especially France, where he had distinguished himself in the Tour de France by winning two stages. Wearing a white baseball cap to mask the two scars that brain surgery left on his hairless head, Armstrong answered questions through an interpreter.

In which race did he expect to return to competition? "Any race," he said. "It depends what the doctors say." He returned to this theme later when a television interviewer asked him how long he expected to be away from bicycle racing. "Six months, a year," he said. "Maybe forever. Living is more important than racing."

April 16, 1997
A Rider Chump

The fellow at the other end of the phone identified himself with a laugh as "a rider chump" and said he was in Italy, "just hanging out." It was Lance Armstrong, but a different one. This was not the Armstrong who, as recently as three months before, reported that his cancer was under control and that he was feeling good. He may have felt it then, but he didn't look it or act it.

Now on the phone was the feisty Lance Armstrong, the buoyant one verging on brash.

He was in Europe now to be a tourist and also to deal with some business. First, he had found an apartment in the south of France to use as a base when he resumed European training. Second, the Cofidis sponsor wanted him to show up at a couple of races and press conferences.

He was at the Tour of Flanders classic early in April and Paris–Roubaix the next week and would watch the Flèche Wallonne in Belgium before returning to Texas. The first two races did not mean that much to him, he said. Armstrong never had done well in Flanders and never competed in Paris–Roubaix because it is scheduled a week before the Ardennes classics, the Flèche and Liège–Bastogne–Liège, which rank among his main goals of the season. The year before, he won the Flèche and then finished second in Liège–Bastogne–Liège.

First came the Paris–Roubaix press conferences.

How did he feel? "I feel good, I feel normal." His hair, which he lost during three months of chemotherapy, had grown back. "I've got eyebrows again," he said with some wonder.

Was he training? "I do two, three hours a day, but not very consistently. It's still something I enjoy, riding my bike. But I missed a day yesterday and it meant nothing. Last year, if I had missed a day, I would have been stressed out."

Did he have a date for his return to competition? "No. Not tomorrow. After the Tour de France. Hopefully. It's only April, and it hasn't been that long since I was very, very sick. I want to race, yeah, but I want to live. I'm waiting for the doctors to give me the go-ahead for hard training and hard racing. They would prefer that I hold off for this year."

"He's happy," said his traveling companion and frequent training partner, John Korioth, formerly amateur racing champion of Texas. "He's doing all the things he never had a chance to do before — taking his boat out, going to rock concerts, just seeing the bluebonnets come up. We've got a lot of bluebonnets in Texas, and he hasn't been home in years to watch those flowers bloom."

Armstrong's cell phone rang — it was his friend and former teammate Axel Merckx, who was now riding for the Polti team in Italy. He was not entered in Paris–Roubaix but would be in the Flèche Wallonne. They spoke about this and that for a few minutes. Then Armstrong told him: "Win the Flèche for me."

"Naw," he said quickly, "win it for you."

July 18, 1997
Simply a Spectator

Heralded by the hum of their wheels, the riders of the Tour de France were leaving Andorra, chatting and joking as they do before the daily battle really starts.

On the sidewalk, just before the riders turned a corner and began to pass out of sight, Lance Armstrong had stood, a spectator. This was not his battle now. It has not been since the previous October, when he was told that he had testicular cancer and that it had spread.

He had not ridden in a professional race since then. After months of successful chemotherapy and continuing checkups, he was sitting out the 1997 season because his doctors feared that arduous physical activity at that point might allow the cancer to recur.

Armstrong joined this Tour as a visitor, participating mainly in a ceremony to honor his former teammate Fabio Casartelli, who was killed in a crash in the Pyrenees two years before.

"It's a strange feeling, but I'm comfortable just being a spectator right now," the Texan said while he spent two days with the race. "It's not difficult for me…" He slowed and chose his words carefully — "to come and watch."

Armstrong between careers. This photo was taken during his 1997 visit to the Tour de France. By now, his hair — and his eyebrows, as he pointed out with awe — had grown back.

Even when the thought was that banal, Armstrong was unaccustomedly slow to respond to some questions. Often the reply was full of uncertainty, as he was.

"It's kind of wait and see," he said of his future. "I'm still being monitored every month, and so far, so good."

His blood had last been checked for signs of disease two weeks before in Texas. Early the next month, he would go to Indianapolis for his three-month checkup and tests in depth.

"My doctors have told me to rest this year," he said. "Whatever happens after this year, it's going to happen. I still consider myself a professional cyclist."

He had a deadline to know how long he would retain that status.

"It's October," he said, "a year after I was diagnosed, in line with the checkups and how they go. The doctors pretty much dictate everything. Yeah, they do.

"The further I go there, the more clear my future will be: whether I'll ride again, whether I won't ride again, whether I can ride again."

Being cleared to ride and wanting to do it are two different things, of course. Armstrong knew that a year off his bicycle, except for intermittent training, would not be overcome quickly or easily. Although he had not gained much weight, and looked fit and happy, he said that his muscle mass had turned soft.

Asked if he had brought a bicycle with him to Europe for training rides, he looked amused. No, he said, he left it behind.

"I've been training so hard," he explained with a big, self-mocking smile, "that I have to taper off for a while."

More important, he was watching his health.

"I feel great, super. I really do. I feel better than I did a year ago." And, he continued, he was enjoying life. "I'm having a blast," he said. "I'm doing exactly what I want to do."

That included playing "a lot of golf," traveling for a week in North Carolina with the Wallflowers band, and visiting Spain with his girlfriend. They went to Madrid, San Sebastian, and Pamplona, where they watched the running of the bulls, before joining the Tour. Afterward he would return from Andorra to Madrid and then flying back to Austin.

Armstrong said he was living day to day and long-term at the same time. "Absolutely. When I wake up, I try to live every day fully and all out as best I can, but I'd be lying if I said I didn't think about what I'm going to be doing 10 years from now."

His options were varied. "I have a bit of a financial cushion," he said, "but I don't have the mentality to sit around and do nothing. I'll find something."

Those options included enrolling at the University of Texas, minutes from his home in Austin.

"I've thought about it a lot," he said. "Business is the logical subject. I could also study medicine, because that makes a lot of sense for me, but it takes so long. I wouldn't mind studying law, but probably business.

"It's an option. I have a lot of options, though, and that's a nice position to be in. Riding again is an option, staying involved in cycling is another, with American industry people."

Which sounded best? he was asked.

"None of them sound bad," he replied guardedly.

But which was best?

After a long pause, he said: "Good question. Sneaky too."

He meant that he knew he was being pressed to say whether he preferred to race again.

"I don't know which sounds best. This is an uncertain time for me. I'm kind of floating in terms of my career and my future and my professional life and my health.

"It's really uncertain, so until there's some certainty, I'm not going to force myself to think about the future too much."

Not many hours later, he was standing on the sidewalk in Andorra as the Tour began to whir out of sight, and then he was gone too.

September 6, 1997
Planning His Comeback

After a year away from racing, Lance Armstrong decided that he felt healthy and motivated enough to try to make his comeback in 1998.

"My doctors are extremely optimistic, and they expect a full recovery," said the star rider, who was turning 26 that month and who had undergone two major cancer operations and four weeklong rounds of chemotherapy.

"They're so optimistic, it kind of changed things for me. I'd never seen that with them. Before that, they were very hesitant, very cautious what they said to me. Before, I thought there was a chance it would come back," he continued, referring to the cancer that had spread to his abdomen, lungs and brain. "I was scared. I had absolutely no security."

But, he continued, in his most recent checkup, his doctor told him that "death is totally out of the question, out of the scenario."

So, asked if he was ready to race again, he replied quickly, "Yes, I am. My engine is the same, my endurance, my heart, my lungs are the same. It's just a question of how much I lost in a year off."

A big problem, he admitted, was that he did not have a team for the coming season. "I have to be part of a team, and right now I'm not. Cofidis has given up on me."

Although cancer kept him from competing in the 1997 Liège–Bastogne–Liège, the Belgian fans had not forgotten Armstrong,

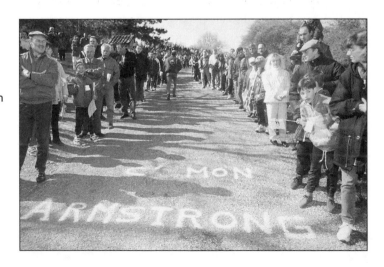

The nominal leader of the Cofidis team, he had a two-year contract through 1998, but it was renegotiated when he became sick. "If I did not race this year, they had the option to drop me," he said. "They think I'm finished. That's great, I love that."

Did he think he was finished? "I think I'm finished with my vacation," he said.

Armstrong revealed that he had offered Cofidis this proposal for next year: He would train at no pay and then compete at a minimum salary, with bonuses for strong performances. "If I started winning again, they would have to pay me my value again," he said. "They turned it down."

His agent was talking with other European teams, Armstrong said, admitting that most teams had already set their rosters for the next year. He said he did not want to ride for a team with many leaders or a team that competed only in the United States.

An obvious choice was the U.S. Postal Service team, which raced a full European schedule and which included riders and officials who had known him throughout his five-year professional career. Armstrong said he had talked with the team and doubted it was interested. "Probably not," he said. "They think I'm damaged goods."

They might, but did he?

"I'm just not sure. I'm very curious about whether I can compete at the highest level again," he said. "That's part of the reason I want to come back, to see if I can do it.

"It also would be great for the cancer community," he continued. "The perception is that once you get cancer, you're never the same afterward. I'd like to prove that wrong."

March 10, 1998
Temporary Setback

Lance Armstrong didn't get very far in the second race of his come-back, dropping out on the first stage of Paris–Nice, but not to worry, team officials said. "A comeback takes time," said Johnny Weltz, the U.S. Postal Team's directeur sportif, citing the extreme cold and strong winds on the course.

In other words, it seemed to be just a bump in the road in what Armstrong called his second career. He called the 1997 season, which he sat out, "a vacation." Armstrong worked on his woeful golf game, traveled with his fiancee, passed medical checkups, spent a week in a musical tour of North Carolina with Jakob Dylan and the Wallflowers, organized a foundation to promote cancer awareness, sat at his home in Texas, and watched the seasons change, even rode his bicycle oc-casionally.

"In '97 I lived the life of a vacationing retired cyclist," he says. "And it was the greatest year of my life. Absolutely."

He was talking before Paris–Nice in a hotel in the remote town of Orgeval, France. A bright lights, big-city guy, Armstrong had hoped to be closer to Paris than this hotel offering little more than a view of the A13 autoroute.

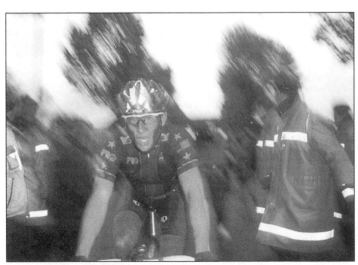

In the 1998 World Championship race in the Netherlands, Armstrong showed that he was back at the top of the sport by finishing fourth.

"Nothing's changed," he grumbled. That was a good sign: In his first career, he often complained about the way bicycle teams are treated by race organizers. It showed he was in form.

In fact, everything had changed. Primarily it was the sight of Armstrong, fresh from his massage and shower, looking lean and race-ready in the casual uniform of the U.S. Postal Service team.

That February, in his first race after an 16-month absence from the sport, he finished a splendid 15th in the Ruta del Sol five-day race in Spain. Not many people expected to see him racing again, especially after he visited the Tour de France that July and told friends how happy he was away from competition. Armstrong had no financial problems, having spent his money conservatively, as he said, and invested it wisely. Why was he racing again? "It was hard to come back," he said, "it was a big sacrifice. Before, cycling was my life and I treated it as such. It was a job, it was a very hard job, and it was something I focused on 100 percent. For a year I just assumed it was gone. So mentally, for 12 months, I learned to move on, to live without cycling.

"Now, to come back, you're reintroduced to how hard it is, to how much focus it takes, how much time you're away from home, how dangerous it is.

"I'm not here for myself," he said, leaning forward in his chair. "I'm not here for the sport, I'm not here to promote cycling in America.

"I'm here for the cancer community. Bottom line. If it wasn't for them and the big question mark that was put on me and the doubt that was put in me, I wouldn't have come back.

"I think there's a lot to prove for a person that's been sick, that's been treated, that's recovering. I'm trying to prove it can be done. It's never been attempted. It's not as if there's been any standard set. It's never been attempted in an endurance-intense sport like cycling. Most people said it couldn't be done.

"I'm healthy, I'm representing a world of cancer patients, families of patients, oncologists, researchers, everything. My situation was bad, very bad, and now I feel wonderful. And the best way to relate that is through my performance."

Those were what he called the positives. There were negatives, too. He was angry that the governing body of the sport stripped him of all the points he earned, dropping him from 1,300 to none, and that few teams were interested in hiring him, since he had no points, which determine the major races a team is invited to. He shifted in his chair, smiled and fluttered his hand. "Ah," he said.

Back to positives. Armstrong was happy with living and training conditions at his new apartment on the Côte d'Azur in France, he would get married May 8 in California, he was excited about the work his cancer-awareness foundation was doing.

Beyond the new season, his plans were uncertain. "I'm certainly not signing now any contract for next year," he said. "I have to decide a lot. First is if I've done everything I set out to do in the second career. The first career, I'm happy. I could walk away from the first career, results-wise. The second career, have I proven to myself and the cancer community that I can be competitive again?

"In a lot of ways, I've already done that at the Ruta del Sol. I can almost stop now. I set out to do what I want to do, and I was a lot closer to packing it in after Ruta del Sol than many people think. Just because I proved it."

June 16, 1998
A Glitch in the Schedule

The schedule was worked out precisely: finish the Tour of Luxembourg, drive for about an hour and a half from that country to the French city of Metz, and catch the last plane to Spain for the next race.

Lance Armstrong missed the plane, though. What he forgot to factor in was the time needed for the ceremony — bouquet, kisses, handshakes, photographs — and the drug test that accompany a victory.

"I won," Armstrong said excitedly by phone. "It worked out. Oh, it feels great."

His ebullience after the four-day Tour of Luxembourg was understandable. The 26-year-old Texan had won some big bicycle races before, but that happened in what he refers to as his prior career. The result in Luxembourg, including a victory in the opening stage, was his first triumph in top-level competition in nearly two years. "It means something, it does, it does," he said of his first race in Europe since his withdrawal from Paris–Nice.

He offered no explanation for that. "I think I've worked out a lot of things" in the three months since, Armstrong said from Metz. After sitting at home in Austin, he went off to North Carolina for a week of riding with Bob Roll, a former teammate, and Chris Carmichael, his former coach and trainer.

"That was just plain old-fashioned riding bikes," he recalled. "That's all we really went to do — call it training, call it bike riding, whatever. We just had a good time, neat company for six hours a day, which isn't easy to do. And it was raining every day. So I figured that if I could do that, ride six hours a day in the rain, then I must want to do it. That's all.

"The main thing I changed between Paris–Nice and the Tour of Luxembourg," he explained, "was my motivation. I was off the bike, out of competition, for a year and a half, and when I came back I expected to be at the same level. And I wasn't. I was competitive, but I wasn't winning. And that was the wrong attitude.

"In Luxembourg, I only wanted to finish the race. That was my only motivation. I learned during that time in North Carolina how much racing meant to me."

During the spring he helped organize a mass ride and a race to benefit his foundation — which grossed more than $1 million in fund-raising to fight urological cancer — was married, and resumed racing in the United States with some creditable results.

"That doesn't really count," he said of the American races. "This is a completely different level. "I'm happier this time around. This feels more right or however I can say it — this feels better than in February. Before Paris–Nice, I thought I could just leave at that point and I did end up leaving. I don't have that feeling now."

He was unable to rank his latest victory among the other milestones in his career, he continued. "It's a different satisfaction. I don't think I can compare this to anything I did in my prior career.

"It feels like a second career and the engine feels like a second engine. My body feels different. But I have returned."

Armstrong would ride next in the Tour of Valencia, followed by a race in Germany, before he returned to the United States just before the Tour de France began. "I'm racing 19 days out of the 23 I'll be here."

He would make no predictions about his results in the rest of his season. "I've won this race, but it's not as if I go to Spain and expect to win there."

So there was no point in wishing him well and hoping that the victory in Luxembourg was the first of many more?

"I won't say I don't hope so too," he replied. "But if it's not, it's not. Today has been great, but I've got to take everything in stride. I just want to go one day at a time."

August 3, 1998
The Tormented Tour

A depleted and demoralized Tour de France reached its finish in Paris in what riders, officials, and observers agreed was a state of crisis for the world's greatest bicycle race and the sport itself.

Their consensus was that the drug scandal that enveloped the three-week race even before it began that July in Dublin had devalued a national icon and would possibly alter the 95-year-old Tour forever.

The scandal had also diminished the afterglow of France's triumph the month before in the soccer World Cup. Instead of a second high, the nation had been confronted by spreading gloom from an unexpected source — its beloved race. The Tour holds a special place in France's heart, attracting an estimated total of 15 million spectators, most of them families, to its roads annually. A billion more are said to watch on global television.

"You can't destroy a myth," insisted Jean-Claude Killy, the 1968 Olympic ski champion who was now president of the Société du Tour de France, the organizers. Nevertheless, there was talk already of a boycott of the 1999 race by foreign teams, with the Spaniards leading the way. Four Spanish and one Italian team quit the 1998 Tour to protest what they regarded as violation of human rights by police investigating the use of illicit performance-enhancing drugs.

The scandal, which is believed to be far from over, overwhelmed the athletic side of the race. Marco Pantani, who became the first Italian in 33 years to win the Tour after he dominated his rivals in the Pyrenees and Alps, was consistently forced off front pages by news of drug raids and rider protests.

There was some wonderful racing, including what will become a legendary stage in the rainy and foggy Alps in which Pantani crushed his main rival, Jan Ullrich, the defending champion. But who would remember it? As Bobby Julich, the American who finished third behind Pantani and Ullrich, said, "10 years down the line you may see an asterisk" next to his result.

The riders deserved better, especially Pantani, who accomplished the rare double victory in the Giro d'Italia and the Tour de France two months apart; Julich, who became the first American since Greg

LeMond in 1990 to mount the final one-two-three victory podium, and Tom Steels, the Belgian sprinter who won four stages.

But they were pushed aside by the unprecedented turmoil, which included the expulsion of the world's top-ranked team, Festina, after its directeur sportif said that he had supplied his riders with illegal drugs. In all, two dozen riders, coaches, team doctors, and masseurs were brought in for judicial questioning, and a quarter of them were charged. Five Festina riders admitted that they practiced doping with the artificial hormone EPO, and the TVM team from the Netherlands was due in a French court to testify in a related case.

Besides those two teams, members of two others had been taken into custody and suspicion had fallen on two more in the Tour's roll of 21 teams. A leading rider, Rodolfo Massi, an Italian with the Casino team from France and the former best climber, had been arrested, and more riders would be heard in court in coming weeks.

The 96 riders remaining of the 198 who started were the smallest total since 1983, when 88 finished what 140 began. The overall mood at the finish was somber, with little of the rider skylarking en route that usually accompanies the last of 21 stages. This time few mugged for the television cameras, wore a hat snatched from a fan or rode backward on their saddles.

The atmosphere was summed up by Frankie Andreu, who said he had been talking a few days ago with Patrick Jonker, a Dutchman with Rabobank. "He said that when he came onto the Champs-Élysées this year, he wouldn't have the same kind of tingling sensation of 'I finished the Tour and accomplished something.'

"It's more like 'We made it to the Champs-Élysées, and now we can get out of here and be done with the race,'" said Andreu, who had finished all seven of the Tours he had entered.

Jean-Marie Leblanc, the director of the race, echoed the feeling. Asked if he was happy that the race had continued despite two strikes by riders and a threat by them to go home before the finish, he said, "Happy? I'm happy only to reach Paris. Otherwise, I'm not happy."

Fan reaction was difficult to gauge, since heavy rains nearly every other day reduced the number of spectators, a fact that could not be laid to indifference. At the finish, the Champs-Élysées seemed as crowded as usual despite more rain and the start that weekend of the nation's four-week summer vacation.

For many, the Tour was still the Tour, a high point of the summer, and they were quick to dismiss the drug scandal.

Graham Jones, a Briton who rode five Tours between 1979 and 1987, follows the race now among the 750 journalists who cover it. Like them also, he judged that the race and the sport were in a crisis, "the biggest we've ever seen in cycling."

"Definitely a crisis," said Jean-Claude Leclercq, a former French national champion who rode five Tours and now worked for Swiss television.

"A pity, a shame, a crisis for all of us," said Eddy Merckx, the Belgian champion who won the Tour five times and now was with the race to watch his son Axel finish 10th overall.

Stephen Roche, the Irishman who won the race in 1988, called this "a very rough time," but thought "some good has to come out of it."

"Everybody admits there's a problem and that cycling has to get its act together," he continued. "That's a good place to begin."

This unanimity cracked when questions were raised about who is to lead the investigation into the use of illegal drugs. Few riders and officials believe in the International Cycling Union, which governs the sport and whose president, Hein Verbruggen, spent the last, tumultuous half of the Tour on vacation in India. Fewer still trusted in the efficiency of the many panels that would be set up or in the government officials who promised tighter laws on drugging.

"From past roundtables and conferences, I'd say nothing's going to happen," Andreu said in a typical comment. "It's so political and it's always the same guys involved, and they want to stay in power. That's their political agenda."

With their investigative power and sophisticated laboratories, the police and the courts appear to many to be the only credible alternative.

"The sport will go on," said Mark Gorski, general manager of the U.S. Postal Service team. "They'll clean out whatever elements need to be cleaned out. If it's taken the French police to do it, then that's what it took."

September 24, 1998
A Rider Reborn

Lance Armstrong had a new philosophy — finish what you start — and, he reported happily, it was working like a charm.

"Armstrong's the man of the year," said longtime rival Laurent Jalabert, the Frenchman who ranked first among the world's racers. After Armstrong finished sixth among 169 riders in a time-trial in the Vuelta à España, Jalabert added: "He's come back from so far down that you can't help but admire him."

"I'm pleased so far," Armstrong said on the phone from Spain, where, somewhat to his surprise, he ranked ninth overall in an extremely demanding three-week Vuelta. "I'm doing pretty good, and I feel very good," he said.

"After two weeks of a big tour, I've never been top 10 before," he added. "I've never been in the front group in big climbs, so for me it's definitely been a success."

The Texan, who turned 27 during the race, had come a long way in his comeback season, including on the medical front: His cancer was in remission and he felt fine. "I wouldn't be here if I didn't," he said.

"He's been quite amazing," said Armstrong's directeur sportif with the U.S. Postal Service team, Johnny Weltz. "He's better now than he was before he got sick. In this race, you've got most of the best climb-

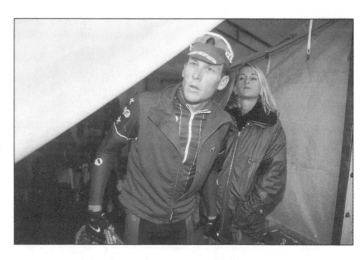

Checking out the weather, with in the background his wife, Kristin, at the 1998 World Championship race.

ers in the world. So if you're up there with them after two weeks of racing, it's because you're climbing very well yourself. It's amazing."

Armstrong brushed off speculation that he had planned to use the Vuelta as a training race for the world championship, dropping out after two of the three weeks.

"I was always planning on doing the full three weeks," he insisted. "After I came back to Europe in July, that was the only goal I set for myself: to finish every race I entered." He had, too, from a fourth place in the Tour of Holland to results back in the pack in the August one-day classics.

Citing the advice of his doctors, he did not compete in the Tour de France in July but continued training in the United States, where he won the Cascade Classic and rode a strong support race to help teammate George Hincapie finish first in the U.S. professional championship.

"At Paris–Nice, I really felt that I left a quitter, and I didn't like that feeling," Armstrong said from Spain. "So I said to myself I can't put any pressure on myself to perform, but I have to finish."

Armstrong had already signed a contract to race again the next year for U.S. Postal Service. "I'm comfortable with this group," he said. "It doesn't have a lot of internal pressure." Otherwise, he was looking ahead only to his honeymoon, probably in the Caribbean late in the fall, which was delayed by his race schedule after his marriage in May.

His remaining races before the season ended late in October included Paris–Tours, the Tour of Lombardy, and especially the world championship in the Netherlands. The course, including 17 climbs of the tiring Cauberg hill, was considered to be tailored for strong riders.

"I've heard it's a good course for me," he said. "I really don't know what's good for me or not. But I plan to be there, and I plan to finish.

"I've finished two world championships," he noted. "One of them I won, and in the other I was seventh. I'm always in the thick of it when I finish." (He finished the Vuelta in fourth place, a performance he matched in both the world championship time-trial and the road race.)

March 10, 1999
Looking for the Sun

Finally, the gray of winter began yielding. In the park, crocuses stood in white rows; down the street, forsythia bushes had flared yellow; on the balcony, the withered jade plant put out green leaves.

Another hint of impending spring was on the road, moving at 40 kilometers an hour (25 miles an hour) along the western flank of Burgundy in a stream of rain-soaked jerseys. That was the Paris–Nice bicycle race, which since its origin in 1933 had subtitled itself "The Race to the Sun."

There is always sun in Nice, the organizers of the race say, even when there isn't. Sometimes at the finish of the weeklong race, after so many promises of sun and gaiety on the Côte d'Azur, almost everybody groans at the sight of more pewter skies. Everybody but the organizers. They are less interested in the weather than in the fact that another Paris–Nice race has ended and now it's time to begin working on the next one.

The organizers are mainly members of the Leulliot family, headed by Josette Leulliot, who took over the sponsoring organization, Monde Six, in 1982 after the death of her father, Jean Leulliot, who began the race.

There are at least three other Leulliots in the organization plus people who have married into the family, and all of them hold day jobs, too — Paris–Nice and the three minor one-day races that Monde Six operates are a passion but not a living for them.

Jacqueline Leulliot, for example, works in a travel agency and has a clause in her contract that gives her a week off every March to head the press office for Paris–Nice. "I do this because I helped my father when he ran the race," she said, "because my family still runs the race and because I love this race."

Since Paris–Nice cannot entice daily television coverage because it cannot afford to share the costs, she comes around at the finish line to show her notes to waiting reporters.

"So and so, number such and such, has attacked and is being chased by so and so, numbers such and such," she says, reading the information that her sister Josette has phoned from the front lines of the 1,354-kilometer-long race. Josette Leulliot is one of the few race directors who, before a daily stage, stroll along the crowd barriers with lists of the starters to distribute to spectators. Jacqueline Leulliot is surely the only press director to meet reporters with a cup of coffee when they come in from a cold, wet stage.

But in an increasingly multinational Europe, where even the currency, the unseen euro, will issue someday from one big vague place, there may not be room for an artisanal race such as Paris–Nice. The year before, the Société du Tour de France let it be known that it was interested in acquiring Paris–Nice and giving the creaky old thing a coat of shellac and modern business techniques, just as it has done for two Belgian races, the Flèche Wallonne and Liège–Bastogne–Liège.

Negotiations were continuing, and the advantages were clear: The Société du Tour de France has the money and the clout to attract the big teams and the star riders who skipped this 66th Paris–Nice. Among the teams not there were Telekom, Banesto, Mercatone Uno and ONCE; among the absent riders was nearly everybody in the top 15, including Laurent Jalabert, the French national champion — a participant in the last 10 editions of Paris–Nice and the winner of the race from 1995 through 1997.

His ONCE team was boycotting the race in its continuing protest over police searches for illegal drugs in the last Tour de France, which the team quit.

"Laurent says that between him and Paris–Nice, it's a love affair," Josette Leulliot has said. "We share that feeling. It's a shame for him. It's a shame that we've gotten to this state."

The Festina Affair, as the drug scandal is known, cost Paris–Nice some of the sponsorship the race needs to meet its 6 million franc ($1 million) budget, she admitted: "We've had to tighten our belts." The overall prize list amounted to just under 800,000 francs, leaving the race far behind its competitors. "Other races are sponsored by newspapers with lots of money," Jacqueline Leulliot said, "or companies with lots of money. We're still just a family business."

For how much longer? "Big fish swallow small fish," she said. "That's the way life is, and that's the way bicycle racing is. Or is becoming."

March 12, 1999
Going Postal

Paris–Nice was not much of a showing for the U.S. Postal Service team, which started with diminished expectations because Lance Armstrong was not seeking his usual fine form in the spring. His training was curtailed during the winter, and he fell in the first stage of the Tour of Valencia and dislocated his right collarbone, forcing him out of that race. When he resumed training outside Nice, his new home away from home, he was knocked down by a French driver, suffering nothing worse than road rash and a $100 charge for the taxi that brought him and his wrecked bicycle home.

After the first stage of Paris–Nice, a short time-trial, Armstrong said that was the only part of the race where he intended to go all out. His reticence would continue into the spring classics, he added. "I'm not going to ride Milan–San Remo at the front, but I'll work for others. I probably won't be anywhere near the front until the end of June." (He was wrong there, finishing second in the Amstel Gold Race late in April after he did most of the work and was too tired to beat Michael Boogerd of Rabobank in the final sprint.)

Why the change in strategy for a rider who usually dominated in the spring? "The team's main objective is the Tour de France, and I work for the team — they pay my salary."

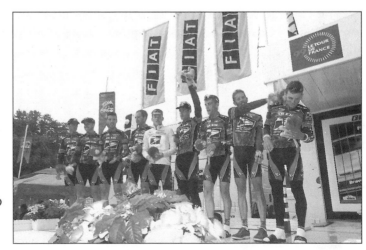

When Armstrong joined the U.S. Postal Service team, few would predict this team would lead the 1999 Tour in the first week.

The Paris–Nice time-trial over 9.5 kilometers left Armstrong happy. "I felt good," he said. "We changed my position this winter, and I was anxious to try that out. I'm riding higher a bit and wider with my elbows, with my hands up higher. It's much more comfortable." Of his ninth place in the time-trial, he added, "I'm both happy with it and surprised by it. The race was really hard, and it's always nice to see that you're not a terrible performer."

He was speaking after the second stage, a rainy and cold one on the road. Referring to the weather, he said, "You know you're in trouble when it's raining on the start line. Can you think of anybody who would have changed jobs with us? Man, it was brutal."

Armstrong noted that he had called his wife to say that the stage was "just like last year, the same kind of day." In 1998, he pulled out of Paris–Nice in rainy and cold weather on the first stage, going home to Texas to rethink his comeback. This time there was no wavering. The weather in the weeklong Paris–Nice turned sunny, even balmy, after a few days of rain, and Armstrong stayed with his program, rode in the pack and ended the race in 61st place out of 103 finishers. That was a far cry from the years when he was finishing second, but he and the team were happy.

Johan Bruyneel, the new U.S. Postal Service directeur sportif, put it in perspective: "Let's say we came to this race with not especially clear ambitions, because Lance is focusing on the Tour de France, like some of the other guys. So we came more for preparation.

"I hope that by the end of March, the beginning of April, we'll be a little better. But our clear ambition is to be at our best in June and July." Didn't Bruyneel call that one right?

March 16, 1999
On the Riviera

"Our goal was to make a home over here," said Kristin Armstrong, surrounded by the beauty of Nice. "It makes things so much more solidified. He travels constantly, so when he comes home, his family's here and a nice home — it makes a big difference, not feeling like a transient. Cohesion and all."

The "he" who travels constantly was, of course, her husband, Lance Armstrong, a resident in Europe during the racing season since 1992. He lived for a couple of years on Lake Como in Italy before he moved to the French Riviera, staying first in different hotels and then renting houses and apartments in towns near Nice, a city of 450,000 on the Mediterranean.

When Armstrong signed with the Postal Service late in 1997, "I figured I'd be here for two years, so I didn't want to rent for two years; I'd rather buy something. Last season we were renting a little house in Villefranche. I'm just anti-rent."

So the Armstrongs began looking for a house to buy. Reading a French real estate magazine during the summer of 1998, he noticed an advertisement for a two-story villa on the eastern heights of Nice, not far from the climb to the Col d'Eze that used to be the time-trial finish of Paris–Nice. The countryside is ideal for training, he said. "If you go inland, it's quieter but hilly." He often rode with other members of his team who live in Nice, such as Frankie Andreu and Kevin Livingston.

"We fell in love with the house when we saw it," Kristin said. "We came to look at it and we made an offer that night. You know Lance: When he wants something, it's pretty much a done deal. Get out of his way."

The house, white stucco and fieldstone, was built on a quiet street in the 1930s with typical Mediterranean flair: high bushes give a small swimming pool privacy from the road, the patio is large enough to hold a big glasstop table and half a dozen chairs, and the yard includes olive, palm, orange, tangerine, and banana trees (basically one of each except for two olive trees). Inside, the house has three bedrooms, two baths, and a big living room that the Armstrongs extended by having two walls removed.

"We just made it more open," he said. "It was a little tight." On a lower level, there is a laundry room with space for a workbench, and a utility room that Armstrong felt could be converted into a wine cellar. The garage held a car, three bicycles, many wheels, and a scooter.

Perhaps best of all is the view, which was spectacular from everywhere on the property. "It's amazing how the view changes, depending on where you are," Armstrong said. "You come up 10 feet or 12 feet and the view totally changes." He was looking out the large window of the master bedroom and over the orange-tile rooftops of his neighbors. "It's kind of hazy today, but you can see the airport at the other end of the city, and you've got the Mediterranean, Antibes, and the mountains back behind." Plus a vast blue sky, which, according to Armstrong, is "even better at night, with all the stars and the lights in the town and the hills."

There was no improving the view, but they felt the house needed some work. "It's an ongoing project," Armstrong said with the practiced voice of a man who had furnished a house in Austin. Work on the new home had been going slower than he hoped, he added with a trace of impatience.

Remodeling work began the November before, when the couple took possession. "The old kitchen, we gutted it," Armstrong said. "The floor, the counters, the cabinets, appliances — everything's new. It's done: They've just got to put the appliances in and hook up the plumbing."

He moved into the living room. "Yesterday, this room was empty, except for the couch and the two chairs," which he bought in 1996. "All the rest was delivered yesterday: the table, the chairs around it, the armoire, the desk." Other furnishings included two small bookcases, a television set, a stereo system, and a few plastic bones for the family dog, Boone, a Maltese. A somewhat calico cat, Chemo, completed the household then.

"The floors used to be ceramic tile and we ripped it out and put in parquet." Armstrong continued. "We also had the house rewired and replumbed. When they ripped out the floors, they found this old plumbing, galvanized steel, and it was going to rust and get nasty, so they replaced it."

Finally, the rooms had been repainted in a light color that he described "off-white, kind of between white and beige and gray. It's warm. The house is a lot warmer now than it was with the tile floors."

"The house wasn't in bad shape," Kristin said, "but it wasn't particularly us. The tiles were mauve-colored with gold, and we really like wood floors."

"I don't know what style the interior of the house is really," Armstrong said. "It's got the same warm feel as the house in Austin, the same colors." Nor could either Armstrong identify the various styles of the furniture except to agree that they worked well together.

"We picked all this out in a complete whirlwind," Kristin said, "so when it all came in yesterday, I was sitting there with my fingers crossed. But I'm really happy with it." When they shopped at stores in nearby Cannes, "a lot of it we just looked at pictures in designer books, so we didn't know the quality until it all came in, because we couldn't touch it or sit on it."

She gave the credit to her husband. "Lance has good ideas. He'll say, 'Yeah, that will work' or 'No, it won't.' He really has a passion for that, a very artistic eye."

June 7, 1999
Italy Grieves

"Pantani, Why?" said the big headline in the Italian newspaper *Corriere dello Sport*, echoing the question that a shocked nation was asking.

There was no immediate answer from the star bicycle racer and national hero. Marco Pantani was in seclusion at home after he failed a blood test and was not allowed to start the next-to-last stage of the country's biggest race, the Giro d'Italia, which he was leading by more than five minutes.

The news that an idol had been disgraced by implications of doping sparked a wave of disillusionment among Italians. But not only Italians.

The embattled sport of bicycle racing this time found itself involved in a scandal that implicated its charismatic leader — then the reigning champion of the Tour de France. If bicycle racing was in trouble, now it was in crisis.

The 29-year-old Italian, the winner in 1998 of the Tour and the Giro — the world's two most important bicycle races — showed a level of 52 percent in the count of red corpuscles in the blood sample he gave to inspectors. The permitted level is 50 percent in tests administered by the sport's governing body, the UCI.

He was immediately barred from competition for at least two weeks.

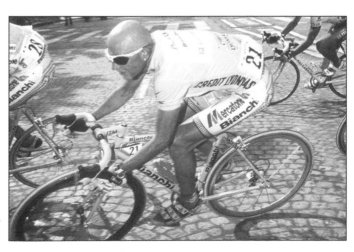

Marco Pantani, winner of the 1998 Tour de France, fell from grace after an excessive level of red blood corpuscles was found in his blood samples.

On the awesome peak of the Gavia, 2,621 meters (8,650 feet) high and a major climb in the Giro, a crowd estimated at 200,000 waited vainly to cheer Pantani on. When the word spread that he had been disqualified, a great sense of anger and sadness swept the fans, according to the French sports newspaper *L'Équipe*.

"For me, it's the end of a dream," said a man identified as Francesco, 65. "He restored a sense of pride to Italy. But that's over now. He tricked us, and I can't forgive him."

Another fan, Andrea, who was wrapped in a pink flag to match the pink jersey that Pantani had worn as the race leader, was equally bitter. "This is a catastrophe for bicycle racing," he said. "Enough! It's all over. What's the point of waiting for the race to come by? Why should I applaud the riders? They're all the same."

The newspaper *La Gazzetta dello Sport*, which organizes the Giro, devoted its first 15 pages to the case. In a front-page editorial that he described as one of the saddest articles he has written, the editor, Candido Cannavo, said: "What hurts me most is the sharp sense of betrayal, on both a human and sporting level. I don't know how far Pantani is to blame or how far he is a victim of shameless provocation, but it's betrayal all the same."

Sounding equally depressed, Jean-Marie Leblanc, head of the Tour de France, said, "We thought everybody understood that times had changed. Obviously not.

"I don't know if this is the fault of Pantani alone or of somebody in his team. I only know that those who did this are irresponsible."

Part IV. Comeback

July 4, 1999
The 86th Tour de France

"It looks good for me," Lance Armstrong said about the short prologue course that opened the 86th Tour de France, and a few hours later he showed just how good it was by winning the race easily.

"Unbelievable," said the leader of the U.S. Postal Service team after he rode with power and authority over the 6.8 kilometers (4 miles) of back road in the Vendée region of western France. "This is just great for the team and for the Tour de France," he said.

"It's obviously been a long year for cycling. As far as I'm concerned, it's history," he added, referring to the drug scandal that shook the bicycle race the summer before and continued with police questioning of dozens of riders throughout the following spring.

"The Tour de France is the greatest race in the world, and the greatest race in the United States too," he continued before heading off to don the yellow jersey of the race's overall leader, the first American since Greg LeMond in 1991 to wear the jersey and to be regarded among the favorites in the Tour de France.

"I know this can be a fantastic example for all cancer patients, all survivors," Armstrong said later. "Life goes on. Hopefully I can prove it's possible to return to a normal, professional life, and maybe I can prove it's possible for you to be better."

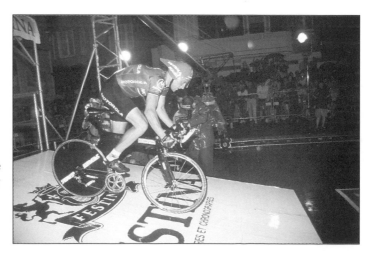

Armstrong starts the 1999 Tour strongly by winning the Prologue. He is shown here at the start of the Prologue — a short time trial.

He was timed in 8 minutes 2 seconds, a speed of 50.7 kilometers an hour (31 miles an hour) on a cool and overcast day. Armstrong finished 7 seconds ahead of Alex Zülle, who also finished second over the course when the 1993 Tour opened here.

"I saw the course in '93 when I did it," Armstrong joked beforehand. "Remember, I'm an old guy." That was his first Tour. He had started five and finished one.

Third among the 180 starters one minute apart in the race against the clock was Abraham Olano, 11 seconds behind. Fourth was Christophe Moreau, a Frenchman with Festina and one of nine riders on that team expelled from the last Tour for drugging. He was 15 seconds behind.

The victory was the first for U.S. Postal in its four appearances in the Tour, and the first time a member had worn the yellow jersey.

Just the month before, Armstrong said that his goal in the Tour was individual stage victories, with a high overall finish secondary. "I'd rather be top 10 with a stage win than top five with a fourth place as my best finish," he said then.

Even before he started the prologue, he reaffirmed this. "Stage victories are still the strategy," he said. "This race is so important to the sponsor in the United States, and we've never had a stage victory. But I've started to think about the overall more."

That was because of his performances the month before in the Dauphiné Libéré and the Route du Sud, two French races in which he demonstrated new power in the mountains.

July 5
Stage One: Wearing Yellow

Two days into the Tour de France, the jury was still out on whether it had retained its popularity with a public weary of doping scandals, but there was no doubt that the victory of Lance Armstrong in the prologue after his battle with cancer was exactly the symbol the race organizers wished for.

Happy? Jean-Marie Leblanc, the Tour's director, was asked before the first of 20 daily stages. He flashed a rare smile in the last year of turmoil and replied: "Yes — for me, for the Tour, and for Lance above all. This is the Tour of renewal, of a return to the top level, and look at him: He incarnates that."

French newspapers echoed that sentiment. The *Journal du Dimanche* said, for example, "The American's success is a valuable symbol. It proves that a serious illness is not necessarily fatal."

The Texan looked splendidly happy (who doesn't?) in the yellow jersey despite heavy rain at the start of the 208-kilometer (129-mile) stage from Montaigu to Challons, a poultry center in western France. As he did after his victory in the prologue, officials of his team emphasized that it would not go all out to keep his jersey in the week of sprinting to come.

"There've been years when we would have killed to defend that jersey," said Dan Osipow, the team's director of operations. "But not now. It's not worth our energy. We'll need that in the Alps." He noted that the winner of each stage got a 20-second bonus deducted from his overall time, which would give a sprinter who did well in the prologue a chance to overtake Armstrong, who would not risk injury in contesting mass sprints.

"If we lose the jersey in the next week," Osipow said, "we aim to get it back in the mountains and keep it then."

Following an early scare, Armstrong did keep the jersey after the first stage, which was watched by big crowds during hours of rain. In the last few kilometers, the sprinters' teams brought everybody together and the victory went to Jaan Kirsipuu, an Estonian with Casino, who finished half a wheel ahead of Tom Steels and Erik Zabel. The winner was timed in 4 hours 56 minutes 18 seconds, a speed of 42 kilometers an hour (26 miles an hour). The pack, including Armstrong, finished in the same time and he continued in the lead by 7 seconds. Kirsipuu, who was 40 seconds behind in the prologue, used his 20-second victory bonus and a smaller one en route to move up to sixth place, 16 seconds down.

The huge numbers of spectators along the roads testified to the continuing, if fragile, place of the Tour in the French national psyche even though the crowd at the prologue seemed smaller than usual. In the starting town of Montaigu, an informal poll — a dozen respondents selected at random with a margin of error of plus or minus 100 percent — indicated that the public was willing to give bicycle racing another chance despite the series of doping scandals. No adverse opinion could be heard because, obviously, anybody who rejected the race would not be found standing in the rain to see it go by.

"It's still a great race and worth watching, even if I don't entirely trust the riders," said a middle-aged man under an umbrella. Hiding in a bus shelter against the squall, a young woman said: "One more scandal and it's all over. Till then, I remain a fan."

Those sentiments were put more elegantly by Alain Delon, the veteran actor, who was a guest of officials at the start. "The Tour," he said, "is part of my childhood, my heritage, part of my life."

July 6, 1999
Stage Two: A Big Crash

What was expected to be a humdrum flat stage, just another showcase for the sprinters, turned instead Monday into a catastrophe for three major contenders, who lost more than six minutes each.

They were Alex Zülle, Ivan Gotti, and Michael Boogerd. All were victims of a crash on a narrow and wet causeway across a bay and never could catch up with a group of 70 riders who made the crossing safely.

"It's a shame that the Tour has to be played out that way," said Zülle, who had finished as high as second in the race.

In a more-expected loss, Lance Armstrong gave up the overall leader's yellow jersey to Jaan Kirsipuu, who made up his 16-second deficit by winning three intermediate sprints and then finishing second across the line in the shipyard city of St. Nazaire.

With 6 seconds deducted from his overall time at each sprint, and 12 seconds for his finish, Kirsipuu now led Armstrong, in second place, by 14 seconds.

Armstrong had hoped to keep the jersey one more day but admitted that the cost of defending it was wearing, nervously and physically, on his teammates. They had to work hard to chase down rivals on breakaways and to stay in high alertness throughout the day.

The Texan said U.S. Postal Service tried to have George Hincapie win the sprints and deprive Kirsipuu of the bonuses, "but he's just too fast right now." Hincapie was third in two of the three sprints.

At the end of the day, it was indeed the sprinters' finish everybody expected.

Tom Steels, the winner of four Tour stages the year before, outsped Kirsipuu and Mario Cipollini, the usual king of the sprinters. Steels was timed in 3 hours 45 minutes 32 seconds, a speed of 46.8 kilometers an hour (29 miles an hour) over the 176 kilometers (109 miles) from Challans.

That speed, stoked by U.S. Postal Service and other teams with yellow jersey dreams, left behind the part of the 180-man pack that was either involved in or trapped behind the crash on the causeway at Kilometer 81.

Known as the Passage du Gois, the two-lane crossing is under Atlantic waters for all but six hours daily, before and after low tide, in good weather, like the overcast and sprinkly conditions of the second stage. In bad weather, it lies so low in the water that is crossable only at dead low tide.

"I knew the passage," said Armstrong, who was in the Tour in 1993 when the road was last used. "But it was just crazy. The slightest wheel movement and you were sliding."

The pack entered the four-kilometer causeway in a long parade that was watched by hundreds of spectators standing barefooted on mudflats where others were gathering shellfish, cockles and mussels, alive, alive-o. Barely a kilometer in, a dozen riders near the midpoint of the pack began falling, and there was no way around them.

"I thought I was well-placed," said Zülle, who has a reputation for being ill-placed, "but I was stopped. Once I got started again I could see the big group in front, but I couldn't make it across to them."

One reason was that the contenders in the front group, including Armstrong, Abraham Olano, Pavel Tonkov, and Bobby Julich realized that they had a chance to leave some formidable rivals far behind and spurred their teammates into hyperspeed.

Forty kilometers later, what had been perhaps a 20-second gap had grown to two minutes. Fifty-six kilometers after that, at the finish, it was 6:03. The chasers must have lost heart, with Zülle, Boogerd and Gotti knowing that their hopes had curdled.

Zülle, one of the Festina Six who confessed to the use of illegal drugs the previous year, now trailed by 6:24. Gotti, the winner of the Giro d'Italia the month before, was 7:04 behind, and Boogerd, fifth in the previous Tour and the winner of the Paris–Nice race that March, was 7:19 behind.

Two riders of the 180 who started the stage did not finish because of the crash on the causeway and one earlier on the landlocked road. They were the homonymic pair of Marc Wauters, a Belgian with Rabobank, and Jonathan Vaughters, an American with U.S. Postal Service. Vaughters, who had been riding exceptionally well and was expected to help Armstrong in the high mountains, was knocked groggy and injured his chin. For safety's sake, his team decided he should drop out and be taken to a hospital to see if he had a concussion.

July 7, 1999
Stage Three: Sweet Dreams

Jay Sweet was a 23-year-old Australian in his first Tour de France who insisted beforehand that he was not intimidated by most of the greatest sprinters in bicycle racing, although in his heart he must have known that he was going to a sword fight armed with a penknife. Then he crashed twice and sprained his left ankle badly.

But Sweet is a sprinter and a good one. Despite his inexperience, the overall weakness of his team, and now his injury, he had the sprinter's qualities of courage and confidence.

"When I crashed the first time yesterday, the pain in my ankle was so, so severe that I thought it was broken," he said. "When the doctor said it wasn't broken, just sprained, I said to myself I'll push on to the finish, I'm not going to let that stop me. Then I went down a second time and I thought it's definitely not my day."

In the starting area of the third stage in Nantes, he brightened.

"But today," he continued, his voice underlining the time element, "is another day, another chance."

It was, but not for Sweet, who finished far back as Tom Steels won his second consecutive sprint. Steels easily finished ahead of Erik Zabel and Stuart O'Grady, an Australian with Credit Agricole. This was the 15th time this year that Zabel had finished second in a sprint, against a handful of victories.

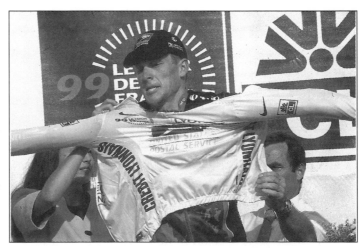

Armstrong slips into just one of his many yellow jerseys, though during much of the flat stages in the first week, he let Jaan Kirsipuu wear yellow.

The winner was timed in 4 hours 29 minutes 27 seconds for the 194.5-kilometer (121-mile) spin over moderately rolling terrain into the likable city of Laval. That was an average speed of 43 kilometers an hour, including a high of 67 km/h in the sprint.

In cool sunshine, the stage past grazing cattle in Brittany's dairy region was watched by enormous crowds from start to finish. So far, the 86th Tour seemed to have kept its hold on the French despite the drug scandal.

Jaan Kirsipuu continued in the yellow jersey, with time bonuses putting Steels into second place by 17 seconds and O'Grady into third by 20 seconds. Lance Armstrong dropped to fourth place.

An unbroken line of 162 of the remaining 177 riders finished in the same time as the winner. Forty seconds behind that pack was Sweet, gamely riding on. The stage the next day was also ideal for sprinters and would offer, as he said, another chance. Speaking earlier about such champions as Steels, Zabel and, above all, Mario Cipollini, Sweet said: "Last year, in the Tour Med, I came within half a wheel of beating Cipo and I came from a long way back too. Since then I haven't raced him, so I've been waiting to have another go."

Cipollini, who was 10th in the third stage and had been blanked so far in the Tour, won four daily stages in the recent Giro d'Italia, or two more than Sweet had won all year.

The Australian's bravado is typical of sprinters, even when they do not have the strong teams that the others have — teams to catch a breakaway and set the stage for a mass sprint or provide a lead-out, letting the sprinter ride in a slipstream and save some of his energy for the final dash.

Teams, moreover, to perhaps impede a rival trying to ride in their leader's slipstream.

"There's a lot of elbowing and pushing and shoving, but there's not much head-butting now," Sweet said. "Jersey grabbing, that's happened to me once or twice, but it's a rare thing."

"Yes," he said slowly. "Cipollini's got such a strong team, Zabel's got a strong team, Steels's got a really strong team."

He left unsaid that his team, Big Mat-Auber, was a French second-division team with a small budget.

"All I need is perfect positioning in the last kilometer," Sweet said. "If I get a look at the finish line, I'll give it my best."

Perfect positioning, however, is not easy to get without some help.

"Definitely not, not when 50 guys all want the same wheel" to follow, he acknowledged.

"If I'm lucky enough to hold the wheel of Cipo, and Saeco is giving him a lead-out, that's the perfect opportunity to maybe go for a stage win, yeah."

In addition to not having a lead-out man, Sweet was also handicapped by the presence of a second sprinter, Christophe Capelle, on Big Mat-Auber.

"Obviously, Capelle and I will try to get organized, but it's difficult. He's going for the win and I'm going for the win. That has advantages too. If he's on the left side of the road and I'm on the right and it's blocked on the left, maybe I can get through on the right. Or vice versa."

"Of course " he added, "we might end up on the same side of the road and both get blocked."

July 7
Stage Four: Where's Cipo?

To all those who had been asking that question, Mario Cipollini gave his answer: In his usual place, crossing the finish line ahead of everybody else.

For the fourth consecutive day, a stage ended in a mass sprint and, for the first time, Cipollini, who is regarded, especially by himself, as the fastest sprinter around, proved it. This time nobody pulled the claws of The Lion King.

Forget his 29th place in the first stage's sprint, third place the next day, and 10th place the day after that. As he explained, "It's not always the best man who wins."

That was then, of course. This was now, and it was different. "I was motivated," he said immediately after he completed the fastest daily stage in the history of the Tour de France. "The team worked perfectly for me and I felt very strong."

He had to be, because Erik Zabel was motivated himself for this stage. The German was celebrating his 29th birthday and desperately wanted the victory. Instead, by half a wheel, Zabel came away with his 16th second place of the season.

Stuart O'Grady was third, followed immediately by nearly all of the 177-man pack, including Jay Sweet in a splendid 10th place.

There was a change atop the overall standings, where Jaan Kirsipuu remained the leader while O'Grady advanced to second place, switching rank with Tom Steels, who dipped to third. Cipollini was timed in 3 hours 51 minutes 45 seconds for the 194.5-kilometer (121-mile) flash from Laval to the Loire Valley city of Blois. That speed, 50.3 kilometers an hour, exceeded the record of 49.4 km/h set in 1993 when Johan Bruyneel, a Belgian who now directed the U.S. Postal Service team, won the Evreux–Amiens stage.

On a chilly day and before another huge crowd, the pack was pushed along by a strong tailwind and covered 52 kilometers in each of the first two hours. Although that speed limited breakaways, 10 riders tried at Kilometer 61 and were left to dangle 20 seconds ahead as the pack refused to slow, and the would-be fugitives could not physically go any faster. The torture ended at Kilometer 91 for eight of them, but Gianpaolo Mondini, an Italian with Cantina Tollo, and Anthony Morin, a Frenchman with La Française des Jeux, persisted.

They, too, were allowed a 20-second lead until the charging pack relented. Off went the two. Mondini, who ranked 158th, 20 minutes 32 seconds behind, and Morin, who ranked 90th, 7:07 behind, were no threats to the overall leaders and so were left free to enjoy the flat countryside that opened before them: the pastures and cornfields of the Mayenne region changing to seas of wheat and the first grapevines of the lower Loire.

Their lead got as high as 6:20 at Kilometer 118 before the top sprinters' teams went to the front of the pack to raise the speed and restore order. By the time the leaders took a left turn and began racing parallel to the Loire River and its many sandbars, the gap was just above three minutes. Down and down it came, with the two caught about six kilometers from the finish. Within sight of Blois's awesome 13th-century château, the pack turned right and crossed a stone bridge into the final kilometer.

In the first three stages, Cipollini's teammates had looked somewhat ragged in organizing a pace for him in what the riders call the Saeco train. This time they got it right and the express went to the front. The Italian roared into the final 500 meters behind two teammates and, as the first dropped off, the second, Gian Matteo Fagnini, provided the leadout slipstream into the last 200 meters. After that, it was up to Cipo.

He pulled hard for the line and Zabel, trying to pass on the Italian's left, could not do it. Some birthday he had.

This was the ninth victory for Cipollini, 32, in six Tours de France and his 123rd in 10 years as a professional. Although the finish was too tight for him to raise his arms in his usual victory benediction for his rivals, there was no doubt that The Lion remained King.

July 8
Stage Five: Questions About Doping

The Festina team was at breakfast, and a quiet breakfast it was. If somebody wanted a platter, he pointed. The nine riders put away plates of spaghetti, omelets, cereal, and ham with barely a grunt and less conversation, like any meal in a bad marriage.

That was Festina a year after the team was expelled from the Tour de France for the systematic use of illegal performance-enhancing drugs. According to other riders and people who know the team, it had split into cliques of those who were new, those who remained and were not involved in the scandal, and those who were and had been reinstated after serving suspensions.

Team members would reluctantly discuss this Tour but not the last one. Nevertheless, the doping scandals that began with the Festina Affair the previous July continued in the sport in general, and this day they briefly edged back into the Tour.

The French sports newspaper *L'Équipe* said that one of four riders tested after the prologue showed excessive traces of corticoids, a banned artificial cortisone, in his urine. Riders are permitted to use corticoids, which treat asthma, among other ailments, if they can offer medical proof that they need them.

The four were identified as Lance Armstrong, Bo Hamburger, a Danish rider for Cantina Tollo, Manuel Beltran, a Spaniard with Banesto, and Joaquim Castelblanco, a Colombian with Kelme. Armstrong was tested routinely as the winner and the others were selected at random. Danish sources said Hamburger had asthma and the appropriate medical certificate.

The UCI later said that nobody had failed the test but that an unidentified rider had exceeded the limit as he had a right to do since he had medical validation.

There went the scandal du jour. The head of the cycling union, Hein Verbruggen, had charged, and the Tour press office had confirmed that the race's press corps of more than 700 had been augmented by nearly 200 reporters who had no experience writing about bicycle racing and were suspected of being along to report on doping.

They must have been disappointed when all 180 riders who started the race passed a blood test designed to detect, by implication, the use of the artificial hormone EPO, the drug of choice in the professional pack and of the ousted Festina riders the year before. That period is over, Festina officials insist. Their riders will rarely say even that much.

"We prefer to let our performance speak for the team," explained Yvon Sanquer, Festina's assistant directeur sportif, who was not with the team the year before. "It's not fair to say that the riders have closed themselves off. But the past is the past. This is a new Festina team and they'll be happy to talk once they've done something to talk about."

That didn't happen during the warm 233.5-kilometer (146-mile) jaunt from the entrancing château town of Bonneval to Amiens, at the other end of the charmometer. The rolling stage past unsuspected fields of wheat west of Paris was won in a sprint finish by Mario Cipollini for the second consecutive day. He finished a bicycle length ahead of Tom Steels, with Jaan Kirsipuu third.

Once again Cipollini was ideally placed by his teammates and had the power to hold off his pursuers and confirm that he remained Super Mario. He and most of the 176-man pack finished in a time of 5 hours 36 minutes 28 seconds, an average speed of 41.6 kilometers an hour, or 9 kilometers an hour slower than the record pace the day before. Kirsipuu continued in the overall leader's yellow jersey, with Steels 17 seconds behind.

The highest placed Festina rider in the sprint was Christophe Moreau, a Frenchman, who finished 12th. His next teammate was 50th.

The previous year, Festina was built around Richard Virenque, four times the Tour's king of the mountains, and featured climbers. Virenque was gone now to Polti in Italy and remained one of three members of that nine-man team not to have admitted using drugs, despite testimony by team officials to the contrary.

Six of the nine riders did confess to the police and served suspensions of six months if they were French, seven months if they were Swiss. Of the six, Laurent Brochard, Didier Rous and Moreau had taken big pay cuts and returned to the French team. Alex Zülle had signed with Banesto in Spain, and Laurent Dufaux and Armin Meier had joined Cipollini at Saeco.

All were in the Tour, rehabilitated. Pascale Hervé, a Frenchman, had not confessed and was barred from the race. Neil Stephens, an Australian, retired and continued to deny knowingly using drugs.

July 9
Stage Six: Sprinter's Heyday

Tom Steels, who had already won two sprints in this Tour de France, badly wanted to win the sixth stage because it ended in the French town of Maubeuge, just across the border from his home in Belgium. Erik Zabel badly wanted to win because he had finished second twice in the last three days and had not won a stage yet. Mario Cipollini badly wanted to win because he had won the previous two days and is insatiable, as all great sprinters are.

In a tumultuous finish, Steels crossed the line first, with Cipollini second and Zabel third. But minutes later, the Belgian was disqualified and placed 172nd because of his aggressive and dangerous tactics. After swerving to cut off Jan Svorada, a Czech with Lampre, Steels dug his right elbow into Cipollini a few times just before the line.

The elbows could be pardoned as a common offense, but the swerve was too blatant a piece of interference.

As a result, Cipollini won for the third consecutive day and Zabel finished second once again. And Jaan Kirsipuu, who wore the yellow jersey, moved up to third, with the bullied Svorada fourth. The winner finished the 171.5-kilometer (106-mile) stage in 4 hours 11 minutes 9 seconds, an average of 40.9 kilometers an hour. Of the 176 riders left, 172 finished in the same time, with Steels placed by the rules at the bottom of the first bunch across.

Kirsipuu remained in the lead for a fifth day, 26 seconds ahead of Cipollini and 38 ahead of Stuart O'Grady.

Steels, who trailed at the start by 17 seconds, had hoped to win the stage and its 20 bonus seconds and vault into the yellow jersey before the almost-home folks. But Kirsipuu won an early intermediate sprint and its six bonus points to thwart Steels's plans. No jersey, no victory — his wife probably burned dinner, too.

On paper, where the race is never run, this was another stage for the sprinters: a warm sun, a rolling course of no particular difficulty and the knowledge that their glory days in the Tour de France rival the half-life of a fruit fly. In two days, the first real challenge of the race, a long time-trial, would exhaust the sprinters, who are more accustomed to going all out for 300 meters than for 56.5 kilometers.

Two days after that, the Tour would enter the Alps, where sprinters are an endangered species. Cipollini, the best of them, had already announced that he had a long-awaited appointment for root canal work in Italy and so would have to withdraw in the shadow of the first peak. Two days left for them, then, and the sprinters made the most of the stage — in Steels's case, too much of it.

In a macabre way, the combat in the sprint was fitting. This sixth stage started in the city of Amiens on the Somme River and swiftly passed into the countryside where trench warfare was at its most fierce, destructive and absurd in World War I. Those rolling fields now planted in potatoes and corn were the staging ground of the Battle of the Somme in Picardy.

In two vast, months-long battles in 1916 and 1918, British and Commonwealth forces suffered more than 419,000 casualties, with 20,000 men killed the first day alone in July 1916. German casualties overall are estimated between 450,000 and 680,000. The land taken, lost, and recaptured amounted to no more than a few kilometers along the broad front in what was then known as Flanders before it became the department of the North.

Some trenches are still there in the fields, preserved for tourists. As the riders passed through the sunny countryside they might have noticed at least one World War I memorial plinth erected on the edge of a field or the statues in many villages of a soldier, his rifle and bayonet pointing at the sky and the names of the dead filling all sides of the huge stone on which he stood.

July 10
Stage Seven: Cipo's Fourth

Mario Cipollini closed out a glorious week by winning his fourth consecutive stage, equaling a feat last accomplished in 1930.

"This is something unreal," he said after thanking his teammates for once more providing him with perfect position.

"Unreal" was a good word for it. Cipollini won the day before on a disqualification and benefited on the seventh stage when a rival's foot came out of his pedal, halting him in the last 150 meters. But Cipo looked as if he would have won no matter what. He crossed the finish line with a lead big enough to allow him to raise his arms in his stylized blessing/victory claim and then looked back in interest to see who was second.

It was Stuart O'Grady, not Erik Zabel, the jinxed German with Telekom. After he crashed in mid-race and tore up his right knee and chin, Zabel seemed to have trouble getting his left shoe and its cleat back into his pedal. In the mass rush to the finish, that shoe came out, followed by the right one, causing Zabel to skid but somehow stay upright with both legs dangling like a small boy learning to ride a tricycle. The German finished 27th.

Mario the Magnificent was timed in 5 hours 26 minutes 59 seconds, a speed of 41.6 kilometers an hour (26 miles an hour), for the 227 kilometer stage from Avesnes-sur-Helpe to Thionville. All but

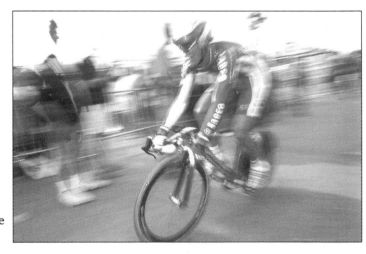

With four stage wins, Italy's Mario Cipollini was once again the king of the sprinters.

three riders among the 176 finished in the same time on a muggy day before continuingly large crowds.

Jaan Kirsipuu, who was third in the sprint, continued in the overall leader's yellow jersey by 14 seconds over Cipollini and 34 seconds over O'Grady.

The four consecutive victories equaled the feat of Charles Pelissier, a Frenchman, in 1930. The record in the Tour de France is five, set by François Faber of Luxembourg in 1909. Faber raced the astonishing distance of 1,623 kilometers, or double Cipollini's total, without losing.

The Italian did not have a chance of tying the record since the next stage was an individual race against the clock for 56.5 kilometers. time-trialing is not Cipollini's forte, nor are the mountains that began two days later.

His victory was another team effort. In addition to giving him a perfect leadout for the sprint, his Saeco colleagues worked hard at the front of the pack to overtake two breakaways, Lylian Lebreton, a Frenchman with Big Mat-Auber, and Jacky Durand, a Frenchman with Lotto.

Lebreton went off at Kilometer 24 with another Frenchman, Stephen Heulot of La Française des Jeux, then carried on alone when Heulot decided 60 kilometers later that the pack was chasing them at such a high speed that the attack could not succeed.

Durand then left the pack and made up the gap of 5 minutes 30 seconds with Lebreton at Kilometer 170. The kamikaze pair rode on and got as far as 8:25 ahead before Saeco, Telekom, and Mapei riders organized the pursuit, which reached them with four kilometers to go.

After that, it was a mad dash into Thionville and Cipollini's fourth sprint victory, the same number he recorded in the Giro d'Italia a month before.

July 11
Stage Eight: Regaining Yellow

Lance Armstrong proved that he could ride a long distance with the same power and purpose that he could ride a short one, winning the Tour de France's first extended time-trial as easily as he won the brief prologue and taking a giant step toward overall victory.

Although there were two weeks left in the race and his credentials in the highest Alps and Pyrenees were still to be proven, Armstrong regained the leader's jersey with a gap of more than two minutes over the field and four minutes over the men who were considered to be his main rivals.

He seemed optimistic. "My advisers told me before the Tour to expect to be stronger in the mountains than in the time-trials," he said.

If that was so, Armstrong was sitting pretty. He crushed the rest of the 176-man field over 56.5 kilometers (35 miles) of twisty and rolling roads. Riding alone against the clock, he caught and passed a handful of riders who started two minutes apart before him, including Abraham Olano, the world champion in the time-trial.

Armstrong rode to victory in one hour 8 minutes 36 seconds or 58 seconds faster than the second-placed rider, Alex Zülle, and 2:05 ahead of Christophe Moreau in third place. Olano was fourth and another American, Tyler Hamilton, was fifth.

The race's new leader was 2:20 ahead of Moreau in second place and 2:33 ahead of Olano in third.

"It was very long and very difficult," Armstrong said after he finished, treading gingerly in his basic French during a television interview. "I'm very happy and very tired. It's one of the great victories of my life."

Mixed with the jubilation in the U.S. Postal Service camp, however, was a sense of caution. "We were confident," said the team's general manager, Mark Gorski, "but you never can be sure. Look what happened to Bobby."

He was referring to Bobby Julich, the American leader of the Cofidis team and the third-place finisher in the previous Tour. Julich crashed badly on a rapid descent and had to quit the race before he was taken by ambulance to a hospital in Metz.

Armstrong was upbeat before the race. "The course seems to suit me well," he said, "but it's not easy." He rode it twice in April on a reconnaissance visit. "It's got several hills, technical downhills, fast and curvy."

He rode the course again the morning of the time-trial and returned to his hotel to warn his teammates about the curve where Julich later crashed. "I told them that it was a tempting descent, very fast, but there's a sharp left turn that you had to be careful about."

Under a warm sun and before tens of thousands of spectators, he handled all the curves with fluidity. Armstrong was the fastest man through intermediate timing points, bettering Zülle's previous best times at three of them. He caught and passed Olano, who left two minutes before him, halfway through the race. The Spaniard had also crashed, swinging far too wide to the right on a lefthand turn and hitting some bales of hay put at the corner as a protective measure. After tumbling onto the bales, Olano quickly righted himself and rode on, but must have been rattled if not hurt.

Armstrong's victory was watched by his wife, Kristin, who was visiting from their home in Nice for the day and posted the flag of Texas in his warmup area. Before Armstrong set out, he gave her and their puffy white dog, Boone, farewell kisses.

More helpful to his victory than the smooching was the collaboration of Hamilton, 28, who started more than three hours ahead of his team leader.

Although Hamilton finished second in the first time-trial in the last Tour, team strategy initially called for him not to ride this stage all out.

But late the day before, that strategy was changed.

"We decided I'd do the first half hard and we'd time every kilometer for Lance," he said after he finished. "After the first half," Hamilton continued, "they said if I was doing well, I could keep going." He was doing very well indeed.

July 13
Stage Nine: Into the Alps

Lance Armstrong opened the defense of his yellow jersey in the best possible way, as he demolished the field and won the first stage in the Alps, put even more time between him and his rivals, and showed that he was the man to beat — if anybody could.

"I think before today there were some questions about my abilities in the mountains, so I think it was important to show that the team and I are strong in the mountains " he said after his easy victory over five climbs and 213.5 kilometers (132.5 miles) from France to Sestrière, Italy.

He said he had surprised even himself with his show of strength. Not an overwhelming climber in earlier years, he had worked at his power and lost a few pounds to help get over peaks.

Was the race over with nearly two weeks to go before the finish in Paris on June 25?

"No, no," Armstrong replied. "I'm still nervous. We don't think we have the race won at all.

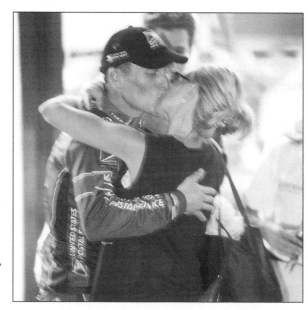

Armstrong hugs his wife, Kristin, after winning the Metz time trial.

"My rivals still have three or four days in the mountains and they're going to be even tougher now. They're all fighters, scrappers, whatever you want to call them."

Whatever, Armstrong finished first by 31 seconds over Alex Zülle, whom he rated as his most dangerous rival. Fernando Escartin, a Spaniard with Kelme, was third, 1 minute 26 seconds behind, the same time as Ivan Gotti, an Italian with Polti, in fourth place.

Two other major rivals were far back — Laurent Dufaux lost 3:30 and Abraham Olano lost 3:10. The Texan widened his lead over the second-place Olano to 6:03, with Christophe Moreau third, 7:44 behind.

Zülle, who lost more than six minutes after a mass crash on the second stage, was fourth, 7:47 behind, and Dufaux was fifth, 8:07 behind.

Those were all big numbers this early in the Tour. Especially interesting, Armstrong said earlier that of the two days in the Alps, he rated his chances much higher on the second day, the race to Alpe d'Huez.

"Alpe d'Huez suits me better because it's harder and more selective," he reckoned, speaking like the master climber he was on the way to Sestrière. When he said it a few days before, though, few knew they were listening to a master.

With a sly grin, Armstrong admitted after the ninth stage that he also said beforeh and that he planned to be conservative in at least the first of two days in the Alps. Then he was one of the first over the major climb of the day, the Galibier pass, found himself without a teammate in the lead group but rode at the front and attacked successfully with about six kilometers to go.

"I did say that about being conservative," he said. "But sometimes the tactics dictate otherwise."

In other words, he said to the field: "Here I am, come and get me if you can."

Nobody could.

Armstrong noted that, although the breakaway group contained three riders for Banesto — including Zülle — and two for Polti — Gotti and Virenque, the French star climber — they all rode not against him but against Olano, who was in a pursuit group a minute behind.

"The other guys just kept pushing the pace to take time out of Olano," he said, and he rode along securely.

He even had a good word for the occasionally drizzly and cold weather high in the Alps, which turned into a downpour just before he crossed the line with his arms upraised.

"This kind of weather makes half the field give up early," he said. "I don't like it myself, but it does make the job easier."

The stage began in the Alpine resort of Le Grand Bornand under overcast skies as an immense crowd of vacationers cheered the riders. The crowd thinned notably atop the Galibier, a climb of 18 kilometers with a grade of 6.9 percent. It is rated beyond category, on a scale mounting from four to one in difficulty. Three of the other climbs were just hills, but the final one to the Italian resort of Sestrière was a toughie, 11 kilometers at a grade of 5.8 percent.

The ramp was awash in tifosi, the Italian bicycle fans, who plastered every rock and fence with signs for their heroes, many of them unknown outside their own kitchens. Who, for example, is the celebrated Fabio Sacchi? (Answer, according to the archives: a 25-year-old rider for Saeco who ranked 168th in the world.)

Among the eight riders who dropped out during the stage were such names as Mario Cipollini, who showed up for the start in Julius Caesar costume, and Jaan Kirsipuu, who wore the yellow jersey most of the previous week until he yielded it to Armstrong after the time-trial.

"I want to keep the yellow jersey as long as possible " said Armstrong. "If that means a day, a week, into Paris — I have no idea."

Increasingly, barring illness or injury, he was alone in that uncertainty.

July 14
Stage 10: Bastille Day

It's all one united Europe now, bound together by open national boundaries and a more or less mythical common currency, so why should French riders in the Tour de Motherland care so much about winning on July 14, Bastille Day, the national day of celebration?

They shouldn't, but they do. Desperately. As they all know, a French victory on Bastille Day can make or revive a career.

But, once again, it was a foreigner who won on the big day, just as it had been a foreigner all but one of the last four years. Once it was even an Uzbek, the year before it was a German, and in 1999 it was an Italian, the unheralded Giuseppe Guerini, who rode for the Telekom team from Germany. He survived a crash with a spectator who stood in the middle of the road with less than a kilometer to go to take a photograph of the approaching leader. The Italian fell, was helped to his feet by the fan, given a pat on the back and a push, and steamed on to victory by 21 seconds.

Pavel Tonkov was second, with Fernando Escartin third, 25 seconds behind. That was the same time as Alex Zülle in fourth place and Lance Armstrong in fifth. The first Frenchman was Richard Virenque in sixth place.

Armstrong, who rode with ease and clarity, received major help from two teammates, Kevin Livingston and Tyler Hamilton. He proved, if there remained any doubters, that he had become a star climber. He also widened his overall advantage. The Texan now led Abraham Olano by 7 minutes 42 seconds, with Zülle third, 5 seconds further behind.

By winning the stage, Guerini registered the first success of this Tour for Telekom, which supplied two of the previous three overall winners in Bjarne Riis and Jan Ullrich. Because of injuries, neither started in 1999.

Guerini finished in 6 hours 42 minutes 31 seconds. That was a speed of 32.8 kilometers an hour (20 miles an hour) over three climbs rated beyond category in difficulty, especially the last 14 kilometers up the 21 hairpin curves to Alpe d'Huez, 1,860 meters (6,100 feet) high.

He was one of a group of seven riders who overtook a Frenchman, Stephane Heulot of the Française des Jeux team, with less than 4 kilometers to go in the 220.5-kilometer 10th stage from Sestrière. Heulot and another Frenchman, Thierry Bourguignon of Big Mat-Auber, attacked together at Kilometer 77, as the 167 starters were descending from the first climb, Mont Cenis. They stayed away for nearly 140 kilometers, visions of sugar plums dancing in their heads as they crossed the Croix de Fer peak. But by the time they reached the Alpe d'Huez ramp, their lead, once over 11 minutes, had shrunk to barely four.

At 36, Bourguignon was too far along to learn to climb now and Heulot left him behind. France's great blue, white, and red hope struggled alone through the many curves, hampered at times by demented fans running alongside him and screaming encouragement and by others flapping French, Spanish, German, and Dutch flags in his path.

The Frenchman worked hard to stay ahead but was overtaken by the handful of top climbers behind him. Heulot finished 11th and Bourguignon 21st.

In the final few kilometers, Zülle, Escartin, and Tonkov each tried to escape and make up some time on Armstrong. He was too alert and strong, however, to let a major rival win that game. When Guerini shot off with about two kilometers to go, the American saw no point in chasing a rider in 14th place, more than 11 minutes behind.

Despite the spectator with the camera, Guerini became the third Italian to win at Alpe d'Huez in four years, following Roberto Conti in 1996 and Marco Pantani the previous two years. Just count it as a victory for One Europe.

July 14
Nasty Rumors

Lance Armstrong had heard the rumors and doubts.

"Innuendo," he bitterly called speculation that he was dominating the Tour de France because he was using illegal drugs.

How else, some of the European press was asking, could somebody who was undergoing chemotherapy for testicular cancer two and a half years before be so dominating now in the world's toughest bicycle race?

He strongly rejected all suspicion. Asked flatly whether he was or had been doping, Armstrong said, "Emphatically and absolutely not."

"I'm not stupid," he continued in an interview as he had dinner at his team's hotel in the mountain resort of Alpe d'Huez. "I've been on my deathbed."

"My story is a success story in the world of cancer," he said, asking why he would jeopardize that. "A lot of people relate to my story. In America, in France, in Europe, they relate to this story."

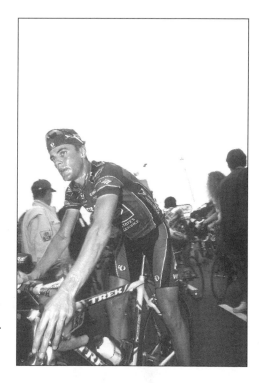

Kevin Livingston was an important support to Armstrong and the U.S. Postal Service team during the mountainous stages of the Tour.

The U.S. Postal Service leader was ahead by nearly eight minutes, he had won three of the 11 daily stages so far: the short prologue, a long time-trial and then the first of two climbing stages in the Alps. He was climbing so powerfully, said teammate Kevin Livingston that he could have won the stage to Alpe d'Huez but did not because he and the team did not want to appear greedy and make enemies among teams that circumstances might cast later as allies.

Speculation about the reasons for Armstrong's performance mounted after the victory in Italy, with veiled references in newspapers and television to the power of a man who had never been known as a dominating climber and who did not return fulltime to racing until May 1998, more than one and a half years after his cancer was diagnosed and treated.

"I've heard the questions and speculation," he said. "The bottom line for me is the same as for Miguel Indurain: Sweat is the secret of my success."

He referred to the Spaniard who won the Tour de France five consecutive times and then retired late in 1996, a man he described as "a good friend and one of my heroes."

"There's no answer other than hard work," Armstrong said. "This team has done more work that anybody else. Look, I'm not going to get mad about the questions because I understand them after the events of last year. I expected this."

He was talking about the drug scandal in the previous Tour and the investigations that had continued in France and Italy since then.

The innuendo bothered him, Armstrong said. "It's bad for the sport, so I can get worked up. It's disturbing for the sport. I think it's unfair." As he worked his way through two plates of risotto for dinner, Armstrong was willing, even eager, to discuss the rumors. Asked if he was taking any medication, he said: "Vitamin C, multivitamins. This is the Tour de France. You need certain recovery products, but certainly nothing illegal."

His defense was considered. He did not repeat his denials, knowing that other riders had made them too and then confessed to drug use under police questioning, but built his case on his record and reputation as a clean rider.

"Who was the world road race champion in 1993, when nobody had heard of EPO?" he asked, rhetorically. "Who? The second-youngest world champion of all time?" The answer? Armstrong, not quite 22.

"Everybody in cycling knows that France is a dangerous place to be," he said, "especially considering that they have extremely aggressive police and the scandal du jour. There are a lot of riders that never, ever come to France.

"But I live in France, I race the whole year in France, my Tour de France preparation was done in France. If I want to dope, that would be ridiculous.

"I'm not a new rider," he said. "I showed my class from the very beginning. I've never focused on the Tour de France before, and when I decided to, I was in France the whole time."

He explained his climbing strength by saying that his focus in the first years of his career had always been on the spring and fall one-day classics.

"At my highest level, though — '93, '94, '95, '96 — when was I tested in the big mountains? I wasn't. It's true," he said. It was "only last year" in the Vuelta à España, another three-week race like the Tour de France, Armstrong said, "when that was an objective. Because of my success in the Vuelta, naturally the team, because the Tour is the biggest race for them, they wanted me to focus on the Tour."

He also credited his climbing skills to a loss of weight, six or seven kilograms (13 or 15 pounds) to his present 158 pounds.

As well-wishers came to his table to congratulate the Texan on his performance, he said that he and his wife, Kristin, would possibly be moving from their home in Nice to another country. "I like Nice. I like France a lot," he said. "But we have people looking through our trash — just bad stuff. The possibility of somebody sabotaging me or pulling some funny business, it's not worth it.

"As Miguel said before the Tour started," he said, referring to Indurain, "you spend 10 years building a career and a reputation, and they can tear it down in 15 seconds. It's scary."

July 15
Stage 11: Transition

Leaving behind the snowy peaks of the Alps, the 160 riders remaining in the Tour de France passed through the darkly wooded hills that fringe the Massif Central, where the race would spend the next four days before it reached the Pyrenees.

These are called transitional stages and they are usually days for the leaders to rest from their labors in the mountains and let smaller fry, men far down in the overall rankings, seek their share of glory.

Seven of the smallest fry — in terms of time behind the overall leader — accepted that invitation. The first was Rik Verbrugghe, a Belgian with the Lotto team, who ranked 96th, one hour 22 minutes 34 seconds behind the yellow jersey when the 11th stage began in Le Bourg d'Oisans, 198.5 kilometers (124 miles) away from its finish in St. Etienne.

Verbrugghe went off alone at Kilometer 80, built a lead of 30 seconds and was joined by five more riders nine kilometers later. They were Dmitri Konyshev and Riccardo Forconi, a Russian and an Italian with Mercatone Uno; Ludo Dierckxsens, a Belgian with Lampre; and Wladimir Belli and Laurent Lefevre, an Italian and a Frenchman with Festina. Later, Alexander Vinokourov, a Kazakh with Casino, linked up.

The game was afoot. The rest of the field slipped into collective lethargy and let the fugitives' lead grow from 2 minutes to a high of 16

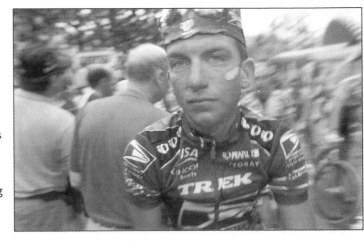

Also Tyler Hamilton was an important support rider for Armstrong and the U.S. Postal team.

minutes. In doing so, the overall leaders had a quiet day and a rare chance to admire the rolling and pretty scenery, including the first serious sighting of fields of sunflowers, always a seminal event in the Tour.

Despite Diercxksens' eventual victory by 1 minute 26 seconds over Konyshev and Vinokourov, and by 22:18 over the pack, nothing changed in the standings at the top. Lance Armstrong remained ahead of Abraham Olano by 7:42, with Alex Zülle 5 seconds further back.

Dierckxsens, who wore the jersey of his country's national champion, left his companions behind about 20 kilometers from the end and sped to victory in St. Etienne. He rose from 77th to 52nd, nearly 52 minutes behind Armstrong.

More significantly, Vinokourov moved from 44th place to 22nd, more than 22 minutes behind. The Kazakh, in his first Tour at age 25, was regarded as a star of the future. A strong climber and the winner of the mountainous Dauphiné Libéré the month before, he floundered badly in the Tour's climbs in the Alps. Perhaps he would do better in the Pyrenees, so it was unlikely that the race's leaders would allow him any further leeway in the transitional stages to come. Vinokourov had moved out of the pool of small fry.

July 16
Stage 12: Simon's Dilemma

François Simon had something that none of his three brothers achieved as professional bicycle racers: the blue, white, and red jersey of the French national champion. But they had something he had not yet achieved: a stage victory in the Tour de France.

The 30-year-old Simon, who rode for the Credit Agricole team, gave it his all and for the third time barely failed to match the victories recorded by his brothers Pascal (1982), Regis (1985), and Jerome (1988). Another brother raced only as an amateur.

"Rats," said Simon, or something like that, after he finished a disappointed second. "I really wanted this victory."

He was 25 seconds behind David Etxebarria, a Spaniard with ONCE, who won the hilly 201.5-kilometer (125-mile) 12th stage from bucolic Saint-Galmier to the perched village of Saint-Flour as the race continued to pass through the Massif Central on its way from the Alps to the Pyrenees.

The winner was timed in 4 hours 53 minutes 50 seconds, or an average speed of 41 kilometers an hour (25 miles an hour) in sunny and warm, but not summery, weather. Huge crowds watched all along the way, as they had done everywhere except atop peaks in the Alps.

With the race's leaders letting low-ranked riders gambol for the second successive day, there was only a small change at the top. Lance Armstrong remained in first place by 7:44 over Abraham Olano, who lost two seconds, and by 7:47 over Alex Zülle.

Etxebarria, a workhorse and promising rider at age 25, rose from 27th place to 15th, or 15 minutes behind Armstrong. The main pack finished more than 12 minutes behind the remnants of an early 14-man breakaway started by Alberto Elli and Massimiliano Lelli. Unhappily for limerick lovers, the two fugitives were not joined by Wladimir Belli.

Heading southwest, the riders transited gorgeous scenery, including endless spruce forests and a succession of charming villages offering the visitor such attractions as a lace museum, a honey palace, and a chance to walk on the world's largest map. Simon had no eye for these distractions; he was committed only to victory.

He won the French championship late the month before, ending a three-year victory drought.

"It's been a while," he said then. "And it becomes a little hard mentally. You keep asking yourself if it will ever happen. But it did, and now I'm not disappointed to have waited for something like this."

An earnest and friendly plugger, Simon had been a professional since 1991 and was the model team rider. He is a decent sprinter and a climber of small hills who won the polka-dot jersey of the Tour's king of the mountains in 1993 by being the fastest up a hill during the prologue. He lost the jersey soon afterward.

He came into the 86th Tour in a stylized tricolor jersey, the colors starting at his shoulders and bleeding down, instead of the usual bands of blue, white and red around the torso. He was also riding a stylized tricolor bicycle.

"I know that in the Tour the fans will recognize this jersey," he said at the start. "I'm ready. You don't know how long I've awaited this moment." Although he had been smilingly posing for photographs and signing any piece of paper thrust at him for nearly two weeks, his thoughts remained on a stage victory.

In his seventh Tour de France, Simon had often finished in the top 10 of a stage — six times the previous year — and was second twice, in 1997 and 1998, before he made it three times on the 12th stage. He said that he would trade his French champion's jersey only for the yellow one. Even then, a brother got there first — Pascal wore it for a few days in 1983.

July 16
An Honored Visitor

Yes, that fellow in the patchwork jersey working his way on a bicycle slowly up the mountain to Alpe d'Huez was Greg LeMond — a graying, more portly LeMond, to be sure, but the same man who nearly secured his victory in the 1986 Tour de France by finishing second there.

The last time, LeMond was racing far ahead of the pack with his only companion his teammate Bernard Hinault. They crossed the finish line with the American's arm over the Frenchman's shoulders in a gesture of brotherhood that lasted only until the next morning, when Hinault announced that he would continue to contest LeMond's lead. LeMond then won the Tour with a fine performance in a time-trial.

Memories of those days are far behind, he said. "I always have mixed feelings when I ride up Alpe d'Huez now, but it's because I'm a poor spectator, and I want to be competing."

What he was doing instead at the Alpine resort, at age 38 and nearly six years after medical problems forced him into retirement as a racer, was leading a dozen cyclotourists in a nine-day visit to France and some of the Tour's daily stages.

"It's a real casual group, ride where you want," said Walt Chapman, an engineer from Cleveland who noted that he bicycled 5,000 to 6,000 miles a year at home. "Greg is there to give us tips and help us learn."

Jorge Jasson, a banker in New York with Chase Manhattan, said, "Greg is the kind of guy that will take the time to give you hints and relate to what you're doing, improve your cycling and, most important, put the emphasis on having a good time."

LeMond always did like to have a good time, to enjoy the food and wine along the way to winning the Tour de France three times, in 1986, '89 and '90. He might have won a few more but — in a similarity to Lance Armstrong's diagnosis of cancer in 1996 — lost more than a season after he was shot and nearly killed in a hunting accident in 1987.

"We were about the same age," LeMond said, "I almost died, he could have died. He went through chemotherapy and major surgery, I went through major surgery. He seems better, but I was never the same afterward. I won the Tour de France twice afterward, but I think on subpar form compared to what I was before that.

"I figure I had three months that went right for me after the hunting accident," three months in which he won the two Tours and a world road race championship. "The rest were just pure suffering, struggling, fatigue, always tired."

"But Lance, it's pretty incredible. He's stronger than he was before his cancer. It's impressive."

LeMond stayed busy back home in Minnesota with his bicycle company and what he termed "miscellaneous products," although he had stopped racing cars, mainly for a lack of sponsors.

He enjoyed leading the bicycle tourists, who paid $12,000 each, not including air fare, for the French visit. "It's fun to let people see the Tour de France and understand it, get them excited about the sport," LeMond said.

It was also fun, he didn't add, to stay at the posh hotel in Grenoble that he favored during his racing visits to Alpe d'Huez, and to eat at the fine Au P'tit Creux restaurant in the resort. Lunch after the climb consisted of an appetizer of preserved eggplant, a mesclun salad, stuffed veal with sage sauce and an apple tart with ice cream and caramelized sugar. As a rider, LeMond was famous for his sweet tooth and love of ice cream, which violated every rule in the old training book before he rewrote it.

Although the group was going home in a few days, LeMond planned to remain and follow the Tour in a car for two stages.

"I've never followed a Tour de France stage in a car," he said. "Last year was my first time back" since the 1993 race. "It was painful to quit. It's a very powerful moment in life, the time when I turned pro and the Tour was my big dream. You achieve part of it, you don't achieve all that you want, and then it's over. You're never going to do it again."

July 17
Stage 13: The Defense Team

The U.S. Postal Service team had spent two uneventful days defending the yellow jersey of its leader, Lance Armstrong. But even on quiet days, the psychological and physical toll was high on a team trying to control the race.

"I'm weary," said Frankie Andreu, who was in his eighth Tour and had never failed to finish one. "I can't wait for the rest day," he added. That would come at the foot of the Pyrenees.

Teammate Tyler Hamilton agreed with him. "Feeling pretty tired," he said. "It's a lot of work at the front of the pack. Of course, it's all worth it. This team is dedicated to keeping Lance in the yellow jersey, whatever it takes."

It did not take much that day. Sixteen riders were allowed to break away at Kilometer 8 (Mile 5) of the 236.5-kilometer 13th stage from St. Flour to Albi. As in the first two of four days' passage from the Alps to the Pyrenees, the 16 riders were all far behind in the overall time standing and no threat to Armstrong. The attack went according to the Postal Service plan.

"The first day we chased down a lot of breaks," Andreu said. When Armstrong's rivals were either caught or discouraged, a bunch of lesser lights was granted free passage. "Yesterday," Andreu continued, "we were too spent to chase much, so we just let them go. Same thing today, I expect."

It was. The 16, who quickly shrank to 15 when one rider could not keep pace, were mainly Italians and Spaniards far down in the rankings. The 15 passed over seven testing hills, up and down all day, until they sighted the red roofs that testify to Albi's Mediterranean orientation.

After 5 hours 52 minutes 45 seconds, the winner was Salvatore Commesso, the Italian national champion and a rider for Saeco, who outsprinted Marco Serpellini, an Italian with Lampre, by two seconds. Third, 2:07 behind, was Mariano Piccolli, another Italian with Lampre. The winner's average time of 40 kilometers an hour was startling in the first heavy heat of the race. For the last 50 kilometers, there was scarcely a house along the race's roads that did not have its shutters closed against the sun.

The leaders' pack finished 22:24 later. Armstrong remained in the lead by 7:44 over Abraham Olano and by 7:47 over Alex Zülle.

Unlike most of his teammates, Armstrong was saucy that morning, for at least three reasons. For one, he usually is. For another, he was comfortable and confident as the Tour's leader. For a third, he did not ride at the very front of the pack, like Andreu, setting the pace. The Texan raced instead in his teammates' slipstream, using about 20 percent less energy than the rider ahead is expending.

Until Armstrong joined the team in 1998, U.S. Postal Service had little experience in controlling a race for a leader. "We did it for Eki in the Dauphiné two years ago," Hamilton said. "Then we did it for Jonathan in the same race last month." He referred to Slava Ekimov, who was a former team leader, and Jonathan Vaughters, who led the Dauphiné for three days before he finished second.

Vaughters quit the Tour after he crashed and injured himself during the second stage. The team lost another of its nine men during the 13th stage when Peter Meinert-Nielsen of Denmark had to abandon because of a damaged knee.

Nevertheless, the overall plan was working. Neither Olano nor Zülle had tried to attack in the four transitional stages, preferring instead to await the mountains. Even when a rider not so low-placed had infiltrated a breakaway and gained time, the American team stayed the course. An example was Stephane Heulot, who ranked 21st, more than 20 minutes behind Armstrong, the day before. He rose to sixth after he was part of an escape and gained more than 11 minutes.

"Heulot doesn't worry us," Andreu said. "He's still nine minutes back, and the way Lance is climbing, he'll take a bundle out of him in the Pyrenees."

July 18
Stage 14: Another Letdown for the French

For more than four and a half hours and 190 kilometers (114 miles), most of France held its breath, wondering if one of their own was finally going to win a stage of the Tour de France after two weeks of domination by Italians, Americans, Estonians, Spaniards and Belgians.

The answer, alas, was "no," and this time it was a Russian. He was Dimitri Konyshev, who rode for the Mercatone Uno team from Italy and who won a two-man sprint finish from Gianni Faresin, an Italian with Mapei, in a lose-lose situation for the French.

The closest a native came to victory was the fifth place registered by Jacky Durand, who had impressive credentials to spark national hopes. A specialist in long-distance breakaways, like the one that day, he was the only Frenchman to win a Tour stage the previous year. He also has been the only Frenchman to win the Tour of Flanders and Paris–Tours classics in decades.

With that history and his reputation as a finisher going for him, Durand should have been a contender in the fourth successive day of long breakaways. He suffered badly with stomach problems in the Alps, however, and had been missing in action since then, as dozens of low-ranked riders like him, but rarely Frenchmen, staged successful escapes.

At the start of the 199-kilometer 14th stage from picturesque Castres to St. Gaudens, Durand looked chipper, much more so than most of the other weary riders. Luckily for them, the second of two rest days was coming up.

"Feeling better," he said, noting he had lost "some opportunities" in the four-day trek from the Alps to the Pyrenees as the leaders proclaimed a truce and let loose the bottom feeders. Durand ranked next to last in the remaining field of 152.

There was no change at the top, as the main pack trailed in more than 13 minutes after Konyshev. He was timed in 4 hours 37 minutes 59 seconds, a speed of 42 kilometers an hour, (26 miles an hour) in muggy weather that turned briefly to rain. Faresin had the same time, with Massimiliano Lelli, four seconds behind in third place.

Lelli, who started one of the earlier breakaways last week with Alberto Elli chose this time as his companion in rhyme Wladimir Belli. Durand and Steffen Wesemann, a German with Telekom, shattered the strophe by riding with them.

Lance Armstrong remained in the overall leader's yellow jersey by 7:44 over Abraham Olano and 7:47 over Alex Zülle.

"I was exhausted near the finish and the Italians worked well together," Durand said later. "I guess this wasn't supposed to be the day when a Frenchman would finally win a stage."

At that point, French riders had no chance to win the Tour itself, something they had not done since 1985. The French press and public were growing increasingly critical and, since the newspapers had nothing to crow about, they had been devoting their vast Tour space (three to seven pages daily) to the possibility of scandal.

First it was the Armstrong drugging innuendos, which had calmed down since he stated flatly in an interview that he did not and had not used illegal performance-enhancing substances. For the last few days, it had been the case of Christophe Bassons, a 25-year-old French rider for the Française des Jeux team who was part of the Festina squad the year before. Bassons was one of three riders there who, team officials said after Festina was expelled from the Tour, did not use drugs.

Since then he had been proclaimed as a symbol of the new rider and even the new Tour. In a newspaper column every day since the race began, he had harped on this, to the point where Armstrong, a strong believer in rehabilitating the sport by not continuing to talk constantly about doping, told him publicly to pipe down.

Bassons especially irritated other riders when he said on television that it was not possible to win a stage simply on talent or class.

Complaining that he was isolated and a target of other riders' criticism, Bassons quit the Tour before the 13th stage. In reaction, the newspaper *Le Parisien*, which ran his column, devoted three pages to the withdrawal.

The 14th stage passed close to Bassons's home in Mazamet and his fans sat by the roadside with black flags. Otherwise, the huge crowds were festive, especially when Durand et al. had a lead of more than 15 minutes. Et al., mainly Konyshev and Faresin, then spoiled the mood for another long day.

July 20
Stage 15: Cementing His Position

Lance Armstrong rode a brilliant tactical race in the 15th stage, then turned on the afterburners and showed that he remained powerful as well as brainy.

He did not win the stage but, barring injury or illness, he sewed up overall victory. With a sly smile, he tried to disagree with that judgment. "The stage tomorrow is long and hard," he said, trying to find reasons not to claim victory.

"But you're optimistic?" he was asked. "I'm always optimistic," he replied, looking like a man without a doubt in the world.

Armstrong declined to contest the final sprint for second place and finished fourth behind Fernando Escartin, Alex Zülle, and Richard Virenque. In the lordly manner of Miguel Indurain, Armstrong's idol, the American dropped back in the last 500 meters and let Zülle and Virenque battle it out.

Escartin had crossed the line 2 minutes and 1 second earlier for his victory. The Spaniard was a strong climber who usually finished in the top 10 in mountain stages but who had never won one in seven previous Tours. He was timed in 5 hours 19 minutes 49 seconds, a speed of 32 kilometers an hour (20 miles an hour) on a sweltering trek over six climbs and 173 kilometers (107 miles) from St. Gaudens to the barren resort of Piau-Engaly, high in the Pyrenees. Crowds were small most of the way along the route.

"I've dreamed of this day," Escartin said. "I've never won a stage before. Is this really my eighth Tour."

He also vaulted from fifth place overall to second, 6:19 behind Armstrong. Zülle remained third, 7:26 behind, as Abraham Olano dropped from second to eighth by losing more than seven minutes to the winner and five minutes to most of the other leaders.

But the day belonged to Armstrong, who used his team and his rivals to perfection. Other Postal Service riders, especially Kevin Livingston and Tyler Hamilton, gave their team leader strong support, while his rivals seemed flummoxed by his coolness and control.

The man in the yellow jersey knew this stage from a reconnaissance he did in May over its six peaks, five of them rated first category and one. None of the climbs was rated beyond category, the most-demanding class.

"We previewed the stage and at the time decided it would be the hardest day of the race," he said beforehand. "It's not as long as Sestrière or Alpe d'Huez," the two Alpine stages. "But with six climbs, it should be decisive."

Early in the day, Armstrong replied to attacks by his opponents, including Escartin, by accelerating and catching them. He rode stony faced, giving away nothing of his physical state. Despite the sweat dripping constantly from his chin, he barely opened his jersey — others rode with theirs unzipped to their waist — and did not pour water over his head although he must have drunk a lake.

He was playing a waiting game, forcing his rivals to choose whether they should do the work of chasing Escartin and Laurent Dufaux, who had opened a lead that, at least on the road, allowed them to overhaul Olano and Zülle in the standings. If Olano and Zülle speeded up, Armstrong would have a free ride behind them; if they stayed put, he would lose no time to them.

On the fifth climb, the Texan accelerated, leaving most of his group behind except for Zülle. When the Swiss faded, Armstrong waited for him, knowing that two men use less energy working together.

On the final 13-kilometer climb to the finish, Armstrong began riding like a man looking for victory. But it was too late to overtake Escartin, and Armstrong was content to ride in with Zülle and Virenque and then allow them free passage.

July 20
No Third Chance

This time they didn't give Jay Sweet a reprieve.

He finished the first Tour de France stage in the Pyrenees the same way he finished the first stage in the Alps — so far behind everybody else that he had to be eliminated, according to the rules, because of the difference in his time and that of the winner.

Rules are rules, the judges said, even though they had the grace not to say that in the Alps. In fairness to them, though, how many second chances does anybody get? Sweet got one, but not a third chance.

"Wish me luck," he said before the 15th stage. The rest day had helped, he added, but his left heel still bothered him. "Maybe it's just bruised, but the team thinks it may be chipped," he said.

In general, Sweet felt less tired, even though he knew that at the end of the day he would be exhausted. He knew that, because he had been exhausted every day for more than a week.

Why was he hanging on, going through all this suffering and sometimes even humiliation? As he said with a laugh, "The only time I get to see the other riders is at the start."

As the Tour's lanterne rouge, the red lantern that used to hang from trains to signify their tail end, Sweet was weary of jokes about whether he intended to defend his jersey. There isn't even a jersey for

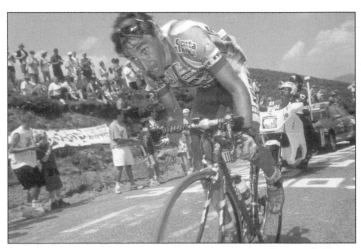

The feisty
Spanish
climber
Fernando
Escartin drives
toward victory
into
Piau-Engaly.

the lowest-ranked rider in the Tour, although there used to be a black one for the last man in the Giro d'Italia.

"Why am I hanging on?" he repeated. "Why not? I've gone through so much already, I might as well keep going. I don't want to give up, I want to finish in Paris.

"I want to finish," he repeated, his voice growing softer.

Sweet, 23 years old, was riding in his second year as a professional for the second-division Big Mat-Auber team from France. For his first Tour de France, he was the last man selected for the team that was given the last nine numbers, which were handed out alphabetically. Sweet wore No. 199, the final number in the race. (He was also tired of jokes about the last number belonging to the last rider, as if it were an omen.)

Most days he rode so far behind that he was alone, with only the handlebars to talk to, as the riders say.

"A lot of times when you're out there on your own, you start asking yourself why and what for," Sweet said. "I guess it's a personal goal," he said. "I mean, this is the Tour de France. The Tour de France is the biggest sporting event in the world, and I'm part of it. I've started it, I want to finish, I'm determined to finish."

That determination carried him through the first time he finished outside the time limit.

Sweet was left behind on the third of six climbs that day in the Alps on the way to Sestrière, Italy. He caught up with a group of stragglers and stayed with them on the descent, then was left behind even by the stragglers on the next climb.

"It was a terrible day," he said, recalling the miserable conditions. "It was raining, it was cold, it was hailing, there was a head wind and I did most of it on my own."

That was for 68 kilometers (42 miles) over three major climbs in one of the heaviest rainstorms people in Sestrière could remember.

"On the last climb to Sestrière, there were no spectators," he said. "Everyone had gone home. The work crews were waiting for me to finish so they could pack everything up. I sprinted the last kilometer, trying to make the time cut. So it wasn't like I was just riding along, enjoying the scenery."

"I was going flat out the whole way to make it. A lot of guys might have given up, but I kept going all the way to the finish.

"At first, I did feel quite sorry for myself and then I said, 'Wake up. Let's get the job done.' Then when it started raining and hailing on me, I actually thought, actually thought there was someone up there making everything as bad as possible. And all I was thinking was 'You're not going to break me, you're not going to break me, I'm going to break this, I'm going to break this.'

"I was three minutes over the time cut," Sweet continued. "The judges said it would be unfair to put me out over three minutes." So he was reinstated.

Perhaps the judges realized that Sweet had accomplished one of the epics of the Tour, like the rider who repaired his broken bicycle at a forge in the early days of the race before World War I, or the rider who gave his wheel to his leader, who had a flat, and then sat on a wall at the side of the road and wept at his lost chance for victory in the 1930s.

Sweet did not see himself in a Tour epic. "This race, it's not going to break me," he repeated. "No one wants to be last, and to keep going when you're last, you gain some respect."

Then he went to ride the first stage in the Pyrenees. He finished 13 minutes outside the time limit, once again sprinting the last kilometer.

Jay Sweet, sweet Jay.

Whatever befell him, and it seemed better not to ask, he left the race with respect gained.

July 21
Stage 16: Le Monde's Quest

Countering accusations in a French newspaper that he had used an illegal drug, Lance Armstrong said that he had treated a rash with a skin cream that contained a banned substance. But he added that "it has absolutely nothing to do with performance," and that "this is not a doping story."

He was supported by the governing body of the sport, which said in a statement that "minimal trace" of a cortisone substance that were found in a test of the American "did not constitute doping."

In a news conference in Pau after the 16th stage, a bitter Armstrong described himself as "persecute" and a victim of "vulture journalism." He singled out the French newspaper *Le Monde*, which had devoted two long articles to Armstrong and drug tests he took in the race's first two days, July 3 and 4.

Discussing the results, the newspaper said that they showed "traces" that did not reveal quantity but did show that he used a banned medication. It identified the product as a glucocorticoid, which it described as "steroid hormones secreted naturally." Armstrong did not identify the salve he used.

"They say stress causes cancer," said Armstrong, alluding to his testicular cancer. "So, if you want to avoid cancer, don't come to the Tour de France and wear the yellow jersey. It's too much stress."

He appeared strained and weary as he spoke. Part of that was due to the long stage over four mountains that he had completed, consolidating his lead, half an hour before. He finished the 16th stage among a small group of leaders, including Alex Zülle and Fernando Escartin, who allowed five minor riders to contest the finish, which was won by David Etxebarria of ONCE.

But the stage result, which sewed up his victory when the Tour reached Paris in a few days, was far from Armstrong's mind now. He was focused on the drug charges.

"I made a mistake in taking something I didn't consider to be a drug " he said, referring to what he called "a topical cream" for a skin rash and saddlesore. "When I think of taking something, I think of pills, inhalers, injections," he continued. "I didn't consider skin cream 'taking something.'"

Defending him, the UCI said that he had used the salve Cemalyt "to treat a skin allergy," and had presented a medical prescription to justify its use. "After discussion with French authorities," the organization continued, "we declare with the greatest firmness that this was a use authorized by the rules and does not therefore constitute doping."

At his news conference, Armstrong was pressed by a reporter for *Le Monde*, an authoritative and respected daily newspaper but one considered to have a bias against the Tour de France. Its reporters had been refused interviews by officials of the U.S. Postal Service team with the explanation that the paper's goals were not those of the team's.

The reporter asked why the race leader denied earlier in the week that he had presented a medical certificate to justify the use of a banned substance.

"Are you calling me a liar or a doper?" Armstrong asked in his only flash of anger. He then said that he had made a mistake.

In response to another question about the speculation that surrounded his domination of the bicycle race after his treatment for cancer, he said that he was tired of questions about "How is that possible?"

His comeback from the illness and his thwarted attempts to find an employer afterward, he continued, had been marked by the same question.

"You have to believe in yourself," he said. "You have to fight, you have to hold the line."

Discussing speculation about his comeback and what Armstrong had described as "innuendo," he said, "It's bad for the sport, for the Tour. and for me.

"I understand why there are more journalists here this year than ever before," he continued, referring to nearly 200 reporters accredited above the usual 750. They were widely thought to be more interested in drug scandals than in the race itself.

"I can understand their interest," Armstrong said, but reporters should be "a little more professional, a little more respectful."

After his news conference, he appeared on a television show devoted to the Tour and was asked briefly about the charges and his defense.

"I'll sleep better tonight," he said.

July 22
Stage 17: Some Attacks

Most of the riders in the Tour de France were weary and looking forward mainly to the end in Paris, which should have meant that the long, flat 17th stage would be raced at a moderate speed by a compact pack. Piano, piano, as the riders say — quietly.

"Don't bet on it," Jens Voigt warned beforehand. "A lot of teams haven't won anything yet, and there aren't many chances left," said the German rider for the Credit Agricole team. "Some people are going to be attacking."

Eight people, to be exact. Representing such have-not teams as Festina, Vitalicio, Lotto, Big Mat-Auber, Française des Jeux and, yes, Credit Agricole, the eight jumped away at Kilometer 45 (Mile 28) of the 200 overcast and breezy kilometers from backwater Mourenx to the wine center of Bordeaux.

Their lead reached a maximum of 7 minutes 55 seconds at Kilometer 100 before a speedy chase began to reel them in. Order was restored with 15 kilometers to go, when the last two fugitives were sopped up.

Then it was the time for the obligatory sprint in Bordeaux, which has welcomed the Tour nearly every year since it started in 1903 and has almost always witnessed a mass finish because of the flat country leading into town.

Tom Steels, an unfamiliar name the last 10 days as the race passed through the mountains and the Massif Central, proved that the wear and tear had not reduced his power. Registering his third victory, he won by half a bicycle length over Robbie McEwen, an Australian with Rabobank. Erik Zabel was third despite thunderous leadout support from his teammates.

Among the top sprinters two years ago, Zabel had obviously lost rapidity in the final 200 meters and was obliged now to settle for second and third places. He was wearing the green points jersey, however, and seemed certain to bear it to Paris for a record fourth successive year.

Lance Armstrong had a quiet day although the pack was disrupted twice — once when firemen protesting something stopped the race shortly after its start and then when a spectator about seven kilometers from the finish hurled a cloud of pepper into the path of the riders, interfering with the vision of some.

The Texan continued to wear the yellow jersey by 6:15 minutes over Fernando Escartin and 7:28 over Alex Zülle.

Despite his early hopes, Voigt was nowhere near that group of leaders. He finished the day in 62nd place among the remaining 141 riders, more than an hour and 45 minutes behind Armstrong. The mountains did him in, which was surprising for a man who usually rides strongly as the road rises.

After he finished a fine eighth in the first long time-trial, the 27-year-old German was optimistic about his overall chances.

Voigt showed no overwhelming disappointment before this stage, possibly because he has dealt with setbacks before. Despite a strong record as a member of Germany's national amateur team, he found it nearly impossible to find a job when he decided to turn professional in 1997.

"I made a little book about me, what races I did and the years, how many kilometers I trained and I sent it to the top 22 teams," he said. "I really put a big effort into it: colors and photographs, and printed on a computer, really nice," he continued. "Then I had it translated into English and French.

"I sent it to the teams and I said, 'Hey, please at least answer me. Say yes or no, but answer me: What's the story?' But only two teams answered, Festina and Rabobank, and both said no."

The Telekom team in Germany was especially uninterested. "I tried three years to get a contract with them, and they never wanted me."

He signed finally with the Giant ZVVZ team in Australia, performed well, and was recommended by officials there to Credit Agricole, then under the colors of the Gan insurance company. In his first season in France in 1998 he rode so well that he was elected third-leading bicycle racer of the year in Germany, behind Zabel and Jan Ullrich, who finished second in the Tour and also rode for Telekom. Earlier in 1999, Voigt won the respected Criterium International in France.

"I think Telekom would like to have me now," Voigt said with a laugh. "Too late. I'm happy where I am."

July 23
Stage 18: In Virenque's Shadow

Amid scattered cries of "la Broche, la Broche," a nickname he despises, Laurent Brochard was making his way to the sign-in for the 18th stage when the air suddenly became aring with air horns, screams and squeals. None of the tumult was meant for Brochard but for the rider who had come up in his wake: Richard Virenque.

Thus it always was. Brochard, a 31-year-old Frenchman who rode for Festina, and Virenque were teammates the last few years on the Festina team.

Virenque was the leader, the winner four times of the Tour's king-of-the-mountains competition, the third-place finisher two years before, and the fans' favorite. Brochard, who wore his hair then in a long ponytail and sported a bandanna over his head, was a good support rider who unexpectedly won the world road race championship in 1997 but was dogged by bad crashes that limited further feats. They were both part of the nine-man team that was expelled from the last Tour.

Although Virenque had not admitted to using illegal drugs, Brochard had, and he served a six-month suspension before he was reinstated by Festina with a 50 percent pay cut. In this Tour, Virenque had won the polka-dot jersey of the best climber again and was once more the darling of the French public, which continued to post signs of support along every route. Brochard resided in 81st place, drew little encouragement from the fans even when the race passed through his native region of the Sarthe, and had accomplished nothing.

Even this day, the last real chance for a Frenchman to win the country's first stage before the grand finale in Paris, la Broche (the "spit," as in a rotisserie) was not part of any attacks, not even the late one by 13 riders that produced a winner. That was Gianpaolo Mondini, who left behind his traveling companions to triumph by three seconds at the end of the 184.5-kilometer (114-mile) stage from the tidy village of Jonzac to the theme park of Futuroscope.

Mondini was timed in 4 hours 17 minutes 43 seconds, a speed of 42 kilometers an hour (26 miles an hour) on a breezy day. The flat stage was watched by crowds so enormous that a visitor hesitated to recycle a peach pit or apple core out of the window of his car in fear of skulling a spectator.

Lance Armstrong remained suave in the yellow jersey, with Fernando Escartin, his nearest challenger, more than six unrecuperable minutes behind.

The start was delayed for the second successive day by a worker protest, this time farmers angry about something. Only Virenque's many fans seem to have no grudge against the Tour, which had tried, unsuccessfully, to ban him. Like Virenque, Brochard was not granting interviews during the Tour. But he did not wear the enigmatic smile that his former leader did — Brochard was stony-faced in his silence. The only sign of individuality was the way he wore his long hair now, in small, tight, beaded braids.

"Forget that part," said Neil Stephens, another former Festina rider, who retired after the expulsion and was one of three members of that nine-man team not to have confessed to doping. "Underneath, he's very timid and a gentleman."

Brochard had had his moments other than the world championship. In the 1996 Tour, he became one of the dozen Frenchman ever to have won the stage on July 14, the national holiday, and in 1993 he was second in the French championship.

The world championship, however, was his apex. When he came home to Le Mans, the mayor presented him with a medal. The city's soccer and basketball teams both asked him to throw out the first ball at their games. His fan club numbered 300. A month after his victory, 2,000 supporters flocked to a rally at a race track near his home to honor him. Brochard talked about a recurrent dream after he won the championship: "I see myself passing the line, my arms raised, I hear the speaker screaming my name, I'm up on the podium, and they're giving me the rainbow-striped jersey. It fits me like a glove."

He was not allowed to ride for France and defend that jersey after the Tour expulsion. For the 18th stage, he was in Festina blue when he crossed the line in 50th place, simply another face in the crowd, and just ahead of Virenque.

July 24
Stage 19: Another First

Good thing Lance Armstrong didn't put his money where his mouth is.

"If I were a betting man," he said before the 19th stage, a long time-trial, "I'd put my money on Zülle. He needs to beat Escartin." That reasoning was sound and even accurate up to a point. Zülle did easily beat Escartin, making up a gap of 1 minute 13 seconds, moving up to second place a day before the Tour ended.

But Armstrong beat Zülle and everybody else, registering his fourth stage victory and third in the three races against the clock. The first was in the prologue, just 6.8 kilometers (4 miles), which he won by 7 seconds over the second-placed Zülle. The second was the 56.5-kilometer ride around Metz, which he won by 58 seconds over the second-placed Zülle.

Over 57 kilometers in and around Futuroscope as a last flourish, Armstrong won by 9 seconds over — who else? — the second-placed Zülle. Why recast a hit show? Armstrong's teammate Tyler Hamilton was third, 1:35 behind the winner in a gutsy showing by a rider who gave his all for his leader in the Alps and Pyrenees.

"I really wanted this victory," Armstrong said afterward. "I didn't start with the same fire I had in Metz, but I wanted to show the yellow jersey today." He showed it to vast crowds that stood in the sun and a strong wind at Futuroscope, a theme park devoted to technology. Armstrong rode like a machine himself, finishing in 1 hour 8 minutes 17 seconds, a speed of 50 kilometers an hour — the legal top speed for a car on the same roads — despite the wind.

That performance increased his overall lead to 7:37 on Zülle and 10:26 on Fernando Escartin in third place.

Beforehand, relaxed and excited at the same time, the Texan lounged in a team trailer and talked about everything that came to mind — except for the fact that the next day he would win the Tour de France. Until the moment that he would pull the final yellow jersey over his head, he refused to refer to more than "my potential victory." Not even the prospect of hundreds of fans who were coming from Texas to cheer him on the Champs-Élysées could budge him from his refusal to claim victory.

"You will be surprised at all the people there on the Champs-Élysées that at the last minute jumped on a plane to Paris from Texas," he said. "Neighbors, friends. To ride the Tour is one thing, to potentially win is another, but to be there on the Champs-Élysées with family and friends and neighbors, that's fantastic.

"And I feel a lot of support from the people of Europe, from the journalists — I do have a lot of friends there — and in the sport also, directors, other riders, other teams' mechanics, soigneurs — they become your colleagues and your friends. It's a dog-eat-dog world, as they all are, and in cycling it's really cutthroat, but people have been supportive.

"I'm excited. I'm ready to get this over with. I'm ready to celebrate with family and friends, I'm ready to have a good time. I've lived like a monk for six months," or since the season began.

In his white team T-shirt and blue sweat pants, he looked remarkably fresh for somebody who was on the verge of completing a three-week trek, often through rain, sometimes through heavy heat. His nose showed red against his face, which was only lightly sunburned because of the peaked cap he customarily wore.

If he looked rested, though, he wasn't. "I don't feel fresh," he said. "I started to feel really tired after Piau–Engaly," the first stage in the Pyrenees, a few days before. "That was two weeks into the race, a rough period for anybody. It was a very hot day and I had the stress after the race of more doping innuendos and I'd worn the jersey for a week — all that was hard for me. Then I suffered more the second day in the Pyrenees than I did the whole rest of the race.

"I had a lot of help from my team," he acknowledged once again. "When we got the jersey and said we would try to defend it, people thought we were crazy, they said this team isn't strong enough. The team proved it could raise its level because we wanted to keep the yellow jersey."

July 25
Stage 20: Homecoming

François Simon had his hair dyed blue, white and red to match his jersey. A rider for the Big Mat-Auber team wore a red bubble on his nose. Hats were snatched off the heads of spectators. Lars Michaelsen of the Française des Jeux team briefly joined a family picnic at the side of the road.

When all the usual last-day hijinks were done in the Tour de France, just about the time the riders left behind the suburbs of Paris and spotted the Eiffel Tower, the race settled down to business. That included the traditional 10 passages of the Champs-Élysées and the equally traditional breakaway attempts followed by the usual mass sprint finish.

The winner was Robbie McEwen, an Australian with the Rabobank team, which previously was invisible in the Tour. Second, for the fourth time, was Erik Zabel, with Silvio Martinelli, an Italian with Polti, third. McEwen covered the 143.5 kilometers (89 miles) from the bean fields of Arpajon to the capital in 3 hours 37 minutes 39 seconds, an average speed of 39.5 kilometers an hour (24.5 miles an hour), completing the fastest Tour de France ever. The average speed of the overall winner, Lance Armstrong, was 40.2 kilometers an hour, exceeding the record of 39.9 km/h set the year before.

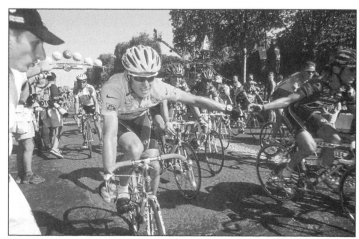

After crossing the final finish line in Paris, Armstrong shakes hands with his teammate Tyler Hamilton, relieved that the 1999 Tour victory is his.

After 22 days, the field of 180 men in 20 teams had been reduced by illness, injury, fatigue, and the rules to 141.

While Armstrong rode off with the grand prize of 2.2 million French francs ($350,000), there were lesser ones in contest too in the big pie of 11.7 million francs.

Zabel won his fourth successive points championship, the green jersey for points accrued at finishes and intermediate sprints. He tied Sean Kelly, the hallowed Irishman, for overall number of victories and set a record for consecutive triumphs. Formerly a paramount sprinter, Zabel had not won a Tour stage in two years and was so upset by his four second-place finishes that he refused to join his teammates in a toast to his green jersey feat. He won 150,000 French francs to share with his teammates, a prize they will certainly drink to again.

Richard Virenque, the controversial French star, won his fifth king of the mountains prize: 150,000 francs and a white jersey with red polka dots. He was closing in on the record of six victories shared by Federico Bahamontes and Lucien van Impe.

The Banesto team was best in total accumulated time, which was worth 200,000 francs, with its Spanish rival, ONCE, second. Benoit Salmon, a Frenchman with Casino, was the top rider under age 25, and Jacky Durand was rated the most aggressive. Each won 100,000 francs.

Otherwise this was a calamitous race for French riders, who failed to win a daily stage for the first time since 1926. The aggressive

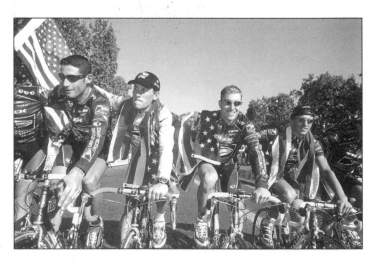

Riding down the Champs Élysées, the U.S. Postal Service team can be satisfied knowing they have helped their leader win the Tour.

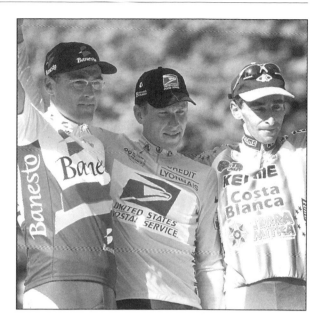

Armstrong stands on the top step of the final Tour de France victory podium, with Fernando Escartin of Spain, riding for the Kelme team, and Alex Zülle of Switzerland, riding for Banesto.

Durand finished last in the overall standings, the fifth Frenchman in five years to do so.

No Frenchman had won the Tour since 1985. The military band that usually serenades the winner with his national anthem would need weeks of rehearsal to play La Marseillaise.

Always a Good Time

A fellow who is crazy for bicycle races (or was crazy for them — since the drug scandals began unfolding, he's not sure) blundered into one the other day. Nothing to it: He walked out his front door on the way to the laundromat and there the race was.

Actually it was the warm-up to the race. Trying to look focused, small groups of riders were coming up the street, turning at the corner and heading west. Small signs announced that a dozen streets would be closed to traffic most of the afternoon to accommodate the bicycle Grand Prix of Suresnes, a town just a few kilometers from the Champs-Élysées but light years away from Paris.

Seventy riders were entered, an official announced over a loud-speaker. Twenty were from the host club, Les Bleues of Suresnes, with a dozen more from its neighboring town, Puteaux. Mysteriously, the team from nearby Rueil-Malmaison did not appear to defend the championship it won the year before. The small crowd behind an opti-mistic number of barriers took this news calmly.

The fellow who is or was crazy about bicycle racing plopped his laundry bag at the curb, sat on a bench and, to pass the time before the start, began to read about the sport in the French weekend papers.

Good news: Patrice Halgand, 25, one of only three Festina riders not accused of systematically using illegal drugs the previous season, won the A Travers le Morbihan race in Brittany. Not much of a race, true, but one of the rare victories this year for what was the world's top-ranked team. More important, according to a reporter from L'Équipe, it was a triumph for health, virtue, pleasure and nobility.

From Germany, more cheer: The unheralded Jimmy Casper cele-brated his 21st birthday by beating Erik Zabel in a stage of the Tour of Germany. "Beating Zabel in a sprint, it's a dream," said Casper, who rides for La Française des Jeux. "I was just a kid when he was winning stages in the Tour de France. If I had known that one day I would beat him." Two days later, Casper did it again.

Good news from Italy: The reason Ivan Quaranta dropped out of the Giro d'Italia after two stage victories was fatigue, as his team said, but fatigue brought on, as it did not say, by a night spent at a disco, celebrating. The 24-year-old Quaranta, who rides for the Italian sec-

ond-division team Mobilvetta, was out dancing until 4 A.M. to mark his victories over Mario Cipollini, the Lion King. Ah youth!

Bad news too: Sixty-seven of the 135 professional French riders showed "metabolic anomalies" in their latest round of health tests. Fifty-four of them had an excess of iron in their blood, often a byproduct of the use of the artificial hormone EPO.

And more: The Casino team in France had suspended Laurent Roux, a fine rider, for failing a drug test administered by the French police. Officials of the Italian Olympic Committee descended on a race in Spain to question Italian riders about drug allegations. The Cofidis team in France reaffirmed its suspension, with pay, of its leader, Frank Vandenbroucke, for failing a drug test.

On the street in Suresnes, the race was ready to start. This was the sport at its most basic, with no team cars, no gangs of mechanics and masseurs, not even a directeur sportif in sight. An official explained that the race consisted of 55 laps in a rectangle through town, a total of 88 kilometers (55 miles), with a cup and a bouquet to be awarded to the winner and the top team. The course was totally protected, he continued, with wardens at each corner to prevent cars from entering. At that moment, a fire truck sounded its siren and raced toward the starting line. The riders made way, smiling.

"It's just a bunch of guys, 17 to 47, out racing," explained one of those guys after he dropped out early. He had plenty of company as heavy heat and continuous attacks wore down the pack. At about the midway point in the race, a group of 10 riders had a minute's lead and managed to keep it.

The group turned the last corner in a rainbow of color and that comforting sound of the whirl of wheels and dashed for the finish line. Far down the Rue de Verdun in Suresnes, somebody held his arms aloft in victory. The loudspeaker announced the winner but his name and club came across in a crackle of sound.

Everybody got to do it all over again the following month when the next-door town of Puteaux presented its Grand Prix. These races are always a good time, even when times are bad.